Praise for
Welcome to the Zipper Club

B RUCE BALLISTER HAS WRITTEN an outstanding book. It chronicles one man's journey from finding out that he had a significant heart problem through the process of diagnosis, treatment and recovery. He does not withhold any details, but instead provides a very accurate and personal account of the entire cardiac surgery process, in an informative and entertaining way.

This book will be of great benefit to anyone who is facing heart surgery. Their family will also benefit from reading it and have a much greater understanding of what their loved one can expect to experience.

I highly recommend *Welcome to the Zipper Club* to any potential heart surgery patient and anyone else who wants a legitimate first-hand account of the cardiac surgery process.

— Jeffery S. Snyder, M.D., FACS
thoracic surgeon

I heartily endorse Bruce Ballister's book, *Welcome to the Zipper Club*. It is a breezy, succinct read of an increasingly common modern terror (heart disease) and what it's like to experience its devastation. His book also covers what it takes to address the disease medically. While the story may be uncomfortable, it is an accurate portrayal, and everyone should read it and then reflect upon how they live, work, eat, rest and play.

— Stephen Michael Hodges
heart surgery survivor

This book brought back a lot of memories. My situation was very similar to the author's in many ways. After my surgery, I was happy to wake up and went through the same things that he did. I enjoyed reading *Welcome to the Zipper Club* and wish it had been available before my operation. This story makes a clinical procedure very real.

— Don Lanham
heart surgery survivor

Welcome to the Zipper Club does a good job of capturing the range of emotions a patient goes through from initial diagnosis of coronary artery disease through the post-surgical rehab required after coronary bypass surgery. Honestly, I thought it was a humorous and thorough explanation of the process.

— Jeremy Fritzsche, FNP-BC
family nurse practitioner

WELCOME
TO THE
ZIPPER
CLUB

Other Books by Bruce Ballister

Dreamland Diaries
Orion's Light
Room for Tomorrow

WELCOME
TO THE
ZIPPER
CLUB

Surviving
Heart Surgery
and Beyond

Bruce Ballister

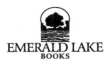

EMERALD LAKE
BOOKS

To my wife Christine and daughter Sarah
my support team who tended to my post-surgery
needs, researched how to solve problems, and were
attentive when I was very much in need of attention.

And to all the medical professionals,
doctors, nurses, EMS techs and support staff
who keep us alive and our hearts beating... Thank you.

Contents

Introduction

I MIGHT HAVE DIED THIS YEAR, or maybe the next. If I was lucky, perhaps not for a couple of years. The exact timing wasn't clear, but all the trend lines pointed to my imminent death from heart disease. I am fortunate—so extremely fortunate—that advice from an Advanced Registered Nurse Practitioner (ARNP) led me onto a path of testing and diagnoses that resulted in a triple bypass operation.

Having gone through that, I'm looking at ten to twenty more years I might not have otherwise enjoyed.

I had retired from full-time employment the year before and was just beginning to transition out of my 8-to-5 obligations into a retired frame of mind, asking myself what single thing I wanted to accomplish each day. It would have been a shame to die so young.

My parents did thirty-odd years ago, when preventive medicine was a new thing and heart surgery was rare. Then and now, a family history of heart disease has been the primary predicting factor for heart attacks.

Due to genetics, some of us are more likely than others to develop hardened or blocked arteries.

I was also more than 35 lbs overweight, which is another primary morbidity factor.

Generally, I felt pretty good—a little more prone to take a break between mowing the yard, a little more likely to lag behind my wife on a bike ride or hike—but I was active, did most of my own home improvements, and considered myself healthy. My cholesterol had been under control for over ten years on Pravastatin. Things were looking up, or so I thought.

But my heart was a beating time bomb that could have gone off at any moment. Several arteries were functioning at only about 20% of their capacity.

I hope this book finds you in seeming good health, before you've had the big one, or maybe after that first tickle scared the bejeezus out of you and sent you looking for more information on heart disease.

There are not a lot of first-person accounts out there. That's why I've written this short docudrama.

This is my story. I hope it informs yours.

Chapter I

November, the Saturday after Thanksgiving

I'M SHOUTING DOWN THE ATTIC STAIRS to the speech-swallowing void that is the garage. I'm hoping my wife is somewhere within hearing range because I need a little more specificity.

Did she want the boxes labeled "Mom's Christmas China" or all of the boxes marked "Mom's China?"

Either way, it means moving more boxes since they were stored expeditiously in the attic last spring when we moved in. Some of the boxes are on the heavy-ish side, and some are so well-packed in bubble wrap that they weigh very little for china boxes—but there are a lot of them.

I shout down again, "Which of the china boxes did you want?" Still no answer.

I turn and set down a box of indeterminate status. A bead of sweat falls from my nose, and I wipe at my

forehead one more time. Yes, it's late November, but Florida hasn't gotten the message, and it's hot up here.

Although there is some minimal decking in the attic storage area, I'm still conscious of stepping as close as possible to the trusses. I've gone through a garage ceiling before. The decking looks adequate to store fairly lightweight boxes and a family's miscellany, but is it up to my 235 lbs?

I find a Rubbermaid tub to sit on and pull the sweat rag from my neck to wipe my brow. Tired. I rub at the stiffness in my left shoulder; I might have pulled something. I shouldn't be this tired in the late morning, but then it's probably over 100°F up here. Listening toward the drop-down ladder for signs of my wife's movement, I realize I need a break, a tall glass of iced tea, and probably an argument to delay this seasonal unpacking event until the evening.

"Hon," I shout into the opening. "I'm coming down."

Rising, I feel a peculiar flash of woozy imbalance. I sit back down. *Wow, it's hotter than I thought.* I take a deep breath, which hurts. I press a palm against my chest. Why does it hurt to breathe deeply?

I try to stand again. My arm tingles—not a funny bone tingle, but a soreness that spreads down and outward from my armpit like the wake of a boat on calm water.

"Ow!" A sharp pain spreads across my chest, radiating outward. No, not radiating, just increasing. I'm suddenly aware of my now rank armpits in a rapid flush of new excretions. Sweat is rolling off my face.

My breathing has become labored. I'm huffing against a wall of muscle that doesn't seem to have the energy it needs. Why are my lungs rebelling?

The world turns sideways. Before I can stop my motion, I've rolled off the Rubbermaid tub and, from my new vantage point inches above the chipboard deck, I can see the outline of the escape route into the garage below. I roll onto my back to ease the pressure on my chest. Pressure? Where did that come from?

This is a heart attack!

I shout again, only no sound comes from the feeble puff of air I manage. Staring at the roof trusses above, I worm toward the opening. Correction: I try to worm toward the opening—to get closer to help, to be heard, to be saved.

My view of the trusses above narrows to a circle and dims. When my wife finds me twenty minutes later, it will be too late.

Not her fault. She had been sorting the decorations that had all known their places in our last house. Where should they be deployed in our new house? Our forever home?

When the EMS crew arrives a few gut-wrenching minutes later, they are fast and professional. They struggle to get my inert mass on a backboard down through the access stair, trying not to let their body language reveal anything. But the unspoken communication in their glances, their quiet reserve, tells my wife the worst.

.••♥••.

Thankfully, this very likely scenario didn't happen. I am writing this while recovering from my triple bypass surgery. The remainder of this book will explain what actually did happen.

I'm not going to pull any punches here. This was all my fault. At least, all the factors that were not genetically related were my fault.

My mother died at sixty-seven, losing a long-term battle with angina.[1] My father, at the tender age of seventy-two, pulled to the side of the road and died of a heart attack.

I knew this. In fact, I had been compiling some of the family history and gathering information to rebuild a lost family tree. So, I knew the age at which they each had died of heart disease. And at sixty-eight, going on sixty-nine, I was in their sweet spot.

Good intentions coupled with a lack of follow-through resulted in the diagnoses of obesity and edema,[2] and possibly congestive heart failure.[3] Each

---

1. Severe constricting pain or sensation of pressure in the chest, often radiating from the lower throat to a shoulder (usually left) and down the arm, resulting from inadequate circulation of blood to the middle layer of the heart, usually caused by coronary disease.

2. Edema is an accumulation of an excessive amount of watery fluid in cells or intercellular tissues, most often a limb.

3. A chronic progressive condition that affects the pumping power of heart muscles.

of these are morbidity factors pointing toward serious heart disease.

By the time of my appointment with my nurse practitioner, my profile—my physical profile—looked like those of a lot of the men around me: pear-shaped. My belly, like those of so many Americans of any age, has been described as a spare tire or, more specifically, a Dunlop—as in, my belly done lopped over my belt. I didn't take too much comfort in being in such a large cohort. I wore extra-large T-shirts at the beach, ostensibly to ward off sun damage, when actually I was ashamed of my gut. At the office or otherwise in public, I wore shirts outside of my belt to flatten my profile.

Despite knowing all the warning signs, possibly buying into a sense of immortality or a mindset of "it won't happen to me," I usually managed to maintain a positive outlook on life. I worked toward and through retirement in a comfortable place with home and family. After all, my wife and I had just moved into our "forever" house. It had an attached apartment into which we had just installed my mother-in-law.

That was supposed to be the big new complication in our lives: caring and providing for a 96-year-old loved one with advancing memory loss. I'd replaced the single hollow core between our living spaces with a pair of solid core doors as sound proofing. At 96, my mom-in-law listens to television at decibel levels near to that of a fleet of semis. We were now contemplating the separation of the air handlers to allow her preferred

84°F from defeating our attempts at summertime temperatures of 74.

In contemplating what was to be my first full summer of retirement, I was looking forward to installing a shelf wall to house the next-size-up flat-screen TV, taking control of a yard that had been ignored for five years and, finally, creating a garage that was a true work space for a hobbyist and home manager. I had just purchased what might be my last vehicle, a top-of-the-line Honda Ridgeline—a truck worth waiting for. The kayaks in the yard were waiting for my wife's retirement a few more years down the road. Things were looking up.

Going in for a stress test was just another step in figuring out what congestive heart failure was all about.

Chapter 2

Diagnoses

M Y LAST ANNUAL CHECKUP with the general practitioner I'd been seeing for over a decade had been several years earlier. My conversations with her had settled into a routine.

Cholesterol imbalance is still an issue, but it's being limited successfully to the high-end-of-safe ranges by 40mg a day of Pravastatin. More exercise will help with my imbalanced LDL/HDL[4] ratio. Weight is still an issue; I need to lose more than a few pounds. I am not morbidly obese at my body mass index[5] (or "BMI"), but I am on the edge of that descriptive statistic.

---

4. The two lipoproteins that react with your cholesterol. Low-density and high-density lipoproteins have different functions. Low-density lipoprotein (LDL) is the "bad one" that carries cholesterol, a fatty compound, to your arteries and contributes to the buildup of plaque known as "atherosclerosis." High-density lipoprotein (HDL) clears cholesterol from your body via the liver.

5. The relationship or ratio of height to weight on a scale that ranges from "underweight" to "obese."

I squirm a bit. "Morbidly obese" sounds bad enough, but for most people, my doctor continues, obesity can be solved by simply losing those extra pounds. My weight at the time was around 230 to 235 lbs, and I've been 5' 11" since I was in my late teens, when I weighed about 185 lbs. Her assessment was taken off a simple wall chart based on average body types.

I find more recently that the National Heart, Lung, and Blood Institute (NHLBI) calculates my BMI as 32.1. On the scale of healthy to unhealthy, I'm obese. (Neither the NHLBI nor the CDC use the term "morbidly obese" any longer.)

My doctor asks to examine an ankle. Pulling down my sock, there are the usual rings that get deeper by the end of each day. They've been there for years.

We continue the discussion about my water retention and the diuretic[6] medication, Spironolactone. I tell her that the meds gave me severe calf cramps while I was sleeping, usually two to three times a night, and I have stopped taking them. With lips pursed in disapproval, she again advises me to stay on the medication and writes a new scrip.

With that, she informs me she's retiring this year and that I should be looking for a new family practice—or do I want to go with her partner? We talk about that possibility.

---

6. An agent that increases the amount of urine excreted.

Handing me the scrip for the medication and smiling, she adds, "And it will help your weight. You probably have 5 or more pounds of water weight."

I'm smiling now. Hey, taking 40mg of Spironolactone will reduce weight and help with my obesity. I leave and don't head next door to the Chick-fil-A drive-thru. I'm not their hugest fan, but they make one of the best drive-thru Oreo milkshakes.

Those good intentions don't last. Going back on the Spironolactone brings back the cramps, and I give up on it after a few weeks. And I don't give up on those Oreo milkshakes.

Nor do I give up on the fast food choices that sustain me on my too-frequent road trips, servicing my consulting accounts. One of my most common trips is a two-hour drive each way to a coastal community with a limited range of restaurant options. That often entails a pit-and-comfort stop halfway and, since it's not polite to use the restroom at a gas station without buying something, I get one of the carb and cholesterol specials and a *diet* coke. Later, on the coast, I don't often spring for the southern seafood salad. I usually opt for McDonald's (it's fast), Subway (it's boring, but I feel good about it), or a Chinese buffet across from City Hall (it's good, but pickled in sodium).

Fast-forward over a year. My primary doctor has retired, and I still haven't researched family doctors

yet. I meet with the ARNP at my retired doctor's office. An advanced registered nurse practitioner has been around a few blocks, and I respect that she's good, especially since I've known Nurse K for years. She is pragmatic and plain-spoken, which I've witnessed several times over the decades.

As in all the major intervals between annual physicals, I've made few changes in my overall exercise routines and still sneak in less-than-healthy foods. But those excursions are usually on the lighter side, a couple of cheeseburgers off the dollar menu and a diet coke. I had stopped getting the obligatory side of fries. I have shunned the heart attack specials at Taco Bell and Hardees for years. I just can't bring myself to consume a double-patty, double-cheese, double-bacon, batter-dipped cardio-bomb, no matter what you called it. And why in hell would anyone eat a taco wrapped in more cheese and another taco?

Our conversation outlines the usual issues as she pokes my ankles. She frowns and pushes into the soft flesh at the base of my shin. Still frowning, she dead-eyes me and says this is supposed to be a very thin covering of flesh over bone. This is pedal edema. I know, I reply, but the Spironolactone gives me horrible leg cramps in the middle of the night, so I've stopped using it. Because, I think, of our long acquaintance (she has seen my wife, daughter and grandson on different occasions), she gives me a look that is a piercing examination of my soul, along with a hint of "you're a simple idiot."

"Look," she responds, "all you need to do is up your potassium levels. Cramping is a well-documented effect of all diuretics, but a banana a day will solve that problem. Or a medium bottle of Gatorade G2." That sounds like a simple enough solution.

But thinking about it, I ask, "What's the big dang deal about swollen ankles? So what? Why is that worth medication?"

This conversation is when the road to recovery begins.

She shakes her head. Surely I've missed something in an earlier interview with the GP. The sympathy-for-the-simple-idiot look resumes. "Have you ever heard of congestive heart failure? You may have it. The edema is a condition, but much more than that, it is an effect and a symptom. If your heart isn't pumping as it should, fluid can build up. And it might just as likely be in your chest cavity as in your legs."

"No, I haven't noticed significant shortness of breath or coughed up spittle anytime recently."

"That's good, but you at least have pedal edema, that's swelling in your ankles." She grasps my hand. "Why aren't you wearing your wedding ring?"

"Well… In hot weather, my fingers swell as the day progresses, and I'd rather wear it for outings than lose it somewhere when I've put it down on one of those days when it became uncomfortable."

She nods her understanding and reaches for my file. It's a fat folder because I've been going to that practice for decades. Then, realizing the answer is in front of

her, she asks me, "How old were your parents when they died, and what did they die of?"

Simplifying the histories, my mother died at sixty-seven after a prolonged struggle with angina. I can still remember rummaging through her purse for pills as she drove through the painful attacks. She was found dead in her bed with a book open on her chest and her thumb holding her spot for eternity. I'm sure she was expecting to just wait out another bout of angina when the real culprit, a heart attack, killed her.

Dad's death is less well-documented, as he was living with an old friend 500 miles away. Our understanding is that he pulled over to the side of the road and died on the spot from a heart attack. He was seventy-two.

She nods. "You're how old?"

"I'm 68, 69 in September."

She writes notes on the daily file summary and looks up, more serious now. "I'd like to refer you to a cardiologist for a stress test."

OK, I'm good with that. I've had one before, but not for more than 25 years as I think about it. Nurse K and I part, and I have another scrip for Spironolactone and new information about how to curb the cramps.

I have since become a fan of Gatorade (though at the time, I could only stomach the lemon/lime variety). By the way, both Gatorade and Powerade have zero-sugar options that I'd recommend.

Chapter 3

Stress Test

I MUST ADMIT to having a go-with-the-flow personality. I suppose I should have done some more Internet research. Like, what is congestive heart failure? What are the implications?

But the good news is, I've been forwarded to a cardiac practice that isn't as overbooked as the largest provider in town. (This may have been because I needed an examination in a hurry.)

Meeting the doctor is a pleasant experience. Only ten or so years younger than I am, Dr. P connects with me on a personal level, and the initial consult results in an immediate sense of trust in his competency. He earns points for wearing pressure socks, which he uses to help control his own edema, but he earns *extra* points for going to Washington, D.C., just to see a concert with the Eagles and James Taylor.

Our consultation is a good one, and I make an appointment for a cardiac stress test.

.₀•●♥●•₀.

I arrive at Regional Hospital's cardiac floor with memories of a stress test administered in my late 30s. I'd been wired for an electrocardiogram and given a strenuous workout on a treadmill. I must have passed because I can't remember any further action. I think, at the time, it was a requirement for the health maintenance organization my employer participated in.

This year's stress test is far more comprehensive. Yes, there is the spaghetti pile of wires going from leads glued to my chest to the EKG[7] machine. The testing starts after establishing a baseline of my heart's performance at rest in a chair. I then move to the treadmill. As the treadmill's speed increases, so does the slope and, as you would expect, my bravado dissolves into a puffing acknowledgment that, yes, I do tire more easily now.

The technical staff says the preliminary reading indicated "reduced perfusion" at 180% of my heart's base rate. They add, "Don't take our word for it. Your cardiologist will give you a full report."

But the staff is not through with me yet. I'm led into a dark room and directed to lie down for a heart ultrasound. Comfortable, cool, dark. I find myself

---

7. A record of the electrical activity of the heart over time. Electrodes are placed on the skin near and around the heart. The printout provides the cardiologist with an indication of when the specific muscle groups of the heart fire and can detect areas of muscle deprived of oxygen. (It's also traced on the machine that flatlines with an eeeeeeeeeeeep when the heart stops.)

thinking I could catch a nap if it weren't for the guy rolling the sensor around my chest from three dozen different angles.

I'm used to the primetime medical dramas' ultrasounds to test a fetus' gender and the rapid *wow, wow, wow, wow* of the sounds generated. I contrast that with the much slower rhythm of my heart—more of a *whoa... whoa... whoa... whoa... whoa.*

I've got to say I'm extremely impressed by the technology investment at Regional Hospital. The technician meticulously measures heart valve function and the valve size when fully opened, and looks for any calcification or other adhesions or abnormalities. I never do get that nap, but on the way back toward the exit, the technician informs me he's been doing this for quite a while and the radiologist will probably confirm that my heart valve function is normal.

I'm feeling pretty good about these two results. The stress test indicates reduced perfusion (translate that to "reduced blood flow") at almost twice my resting heart rate. Sure, why wouldn't I be tired huffing up a steep incline? The ultrasound says there aren't any issues with valve structure or operation.

But the good feeling doesn't last.

A few days later in the cardiologist's office, Dr. P is not as sanguine about the stress test results. The reduced perfusion is not a trivial matter. The results of the

ultrasound are confirmed. Heart valve function is just fine. More testing is needed to determine why there is reduced blood flow and perhaps provide an answer to why I have the resultant edema.

I'm hoping there will be a simple fix, because my edema has been linked since April to the menacing phrase "congestive heart failure." Failure is the key worry-word in that phrase.

In my various realms of experience, failure meant just that: failure. Cool Hand Luke's "What we've got here is failure to communicate" results in his being shot in the neck. The structural supports failed, and the bridge collapsed. I failed a few classes in college due to an ill-timed illness, and those classes required do-overs. A competitive bid failed to yield the company-saving contract, and the company had to shut its doors. Failure always meant a pass/fail level of success. Otherwise, you wouldn't need A's, B's, C's and D minuses.

I understand now that the "failure" in congestive heart failure is a condition caused by a reduced ability of the heart to do its job, which is to maintain the pressures required to move blood through the pulmonary (lung) and aortic (systemic circulatory) systems. The one feeds blood to the lungs for a fresh load of oxygen; the other distributes oxygenated blood to everything else, including itself.

So, congestive heart failure is not pass/fail. A heart attack is pass/fail.

There is a range of experience between the diagnosis of congestive heart failure and a fatal heart attack. But I wasn't there yet in my understanding of the term and of what might be stacking up against me.

Dr. P suggested the next level of testing, which would provide a much clearer understanding of what was going on: heart catheterization. Specifically, this meant inserting a thin tube into the heart and releasing radioactive tracers into the blood stream. The dye tracers provide an excellent image of how the blood is or isn't being distributed into the heart's arterial system.

Chapter 4

Catheterization

THE NEXT STAGE in the escalating and intrusive testing is a left heart catheterization. A small tube will be inserted into a wrist or other available artery, deep enough into the system that its end is located in the left side of the heart. The only pain will be the slight pinch as the incision needle for the catheter, or "cath," is inserted into an artery in my right wrist. There are no nerve cells inside the arteries, so there won't be any discomfort while the cath tube is moving around in the system.

Maybe in the design of Humans 8.0, a little arterial pain sensitivity to calcium deposits would be a good deterrent to continued dietary self-abuse. But I don't think that will happen. Humans are pain averse, but we are also suckers for double-meat cheeseburgers, meat-lover's pizzas and late-night snacks.

The catheterization procedure went more easily than expected, although I don't know what I expected,

which is one of the reasons I'm writing this book: so *you* might know what to expect.

Taken into the prep area, I trade street clothes for a rear-access gown and am reassured multiple times by medical professionals, who do these daily, that I shouldn't worry. Did I look worried? Their joking and casual manner calmed me considerably, and the only pain I noted was the slight prick of the IV connection. There is the promise of a second, later poke by the catheter's lead needle. I repeat my name and birth date at several stages of the prep.

I believe there may have been a sedative administered in that IV, but the best part was the TV. Suspended from the ceiling, on a rig that probably cost 40 or 50 times the cost of your wall mount, is a 60″ flat-panel widescreen TV. Hovering over my chest on a multiple-gimbaled support is an 18″ square box housing the X-ray gun.

Dr. P enters after all preparations are completed. The prep techs had joked that they spend 45 minutes to an hour getting me ready and just as long getting me into street clothes again, but the good doctor can do what he needs to do in ten minutes.

All the equipment in the room is covered in plastic sheeting. To protect it from what I wonder? Bodily fluids? X-rays?

Dr. P is the third or fourth person in the process to confirm my name and date of birth. This has been a consistent go/no-go, pass/fail stage at several steps today.

I pass and get the forewarned "slight pinch" as the catheter needle is inserted into an artery in my wrist just above my right thumb. I am pleased that there is no sensation of the catheter making progress upstream to that wonderful machine we call the heart.

On the widescreen, my heart is thumping away, doing its job at a normal rate. It is not a clear picture of a heart; it is a moving mass in a complex scene in shades of gray. A small tube enters the scene as the catheter moves into position. Those subtly shaded moving gray masses provide enough of a roadmap for the tip of the catheter to enter the entrance to the left descending artery.

On the widescreen floating above, my heart is flexing away, visual proof of the *thadump, thadump* I hear in my ears. A dark cloud of tracer dye swirls in from stage left and moves on.

Dr. P's hands manipulate the probe, and the dyes swirl in again and spread out into the branching arteries. The dark-shaded dyes are quickly pumped into the surrounding tissues, and the artery disappears again into the grey-on-grey image of my beating heart.

It is a genuinely magical moment. The hovering X-ray gun moves to enough angles to get clear shots of the various arteries feeding the heart muscle.

I don't know if you will ever get to this point, but if you do, pay attention. Your doctor has done this before. They are assessing your heart and any visible damage, while making mental and digitally recorded notes as to how to approach an eventual surgery (if you need one).

This whole process is called a "coronary angiogram,"[8] if you want to look it up. It is a digital movie in black and white of the dye tracing procedure.

During that process, your physician may, based on your condition, install a stent,[9] which is a small tube that can open up a restricted artery. This would be discussed with you at the time. In my case, it didn't happen since I needed further work.

While still on the table, Dr. P pulled the X-ray gun out of the way and brought the flat-screen closer. He backed up the recorded angiogram to a point where he could pause and zoom. The screen fills with the dendritic image of my left descending artery. He points to the thick stem of the main artery. "See this area here that's not as thick as the rest?"

I see a section of indeterminate length that I would compare to three lanes of interstate funneling down to one emergency lane—you've probably experienced that. Here, good, plenty of capacity and safety; there, not so good, danger signs on the approaches.

He talks numbers that fly by as my mind grasps the reality. I hear 60%, 70% or, as he points to another still shot, 80%. I finally understand that these are not the percentages left. These are the amount of blockage. So, one or more of those places is 80% blocked.

---

8. Radiograph obtained by angiography (imaging of the circulation of the myocardium by injection of contrast medium, usually by selective catheterization of each coronary artery.)

9. A wire mesh implant inserted via a catheter and expanded inside a clogged artery to improve blood flow.

After the initial pinch of the cath needle being inserted, there are no other sensations during the rest of the procedure. There is a slight warmth when the dye is injected, but no further sensations, even when the catheter was being removed.

Immediately after the procedure, Dr. P talks to my wife and me while in the recovery area. He indicates that, based on these results, he would like to refer me to a cardio-thoracic surgeon. A triple bypass open-chest operation is indicated. In a bit of a shocked fog, we agree and, in only a few more days (the surgeon usually does consults on Tuesdays), we have an appointment with Dr. S.

Chapter 5

Surgical Consult

M Y WIFE AND I ARE IN DR. S'S OFFICE before we have accepted the idea it's actually happening. Dr. P had mentioned that multiple-bypass operations have been performed thousands of times, and the cardiac surgeon he recommended is one of the best in the region. Dr. S tells us there is only a 2% morbidity rate,[10] and a person in my state of health should have nothing to worry about.

I'm not worried, right?

Dr. S looks old enough to have gotten good at cardiac surgery. His credentials, which we'd Googled prior to the visit, seem impressive and include starting new clinics and developing new techniques. He is one of the primary cardiac surgeons at Regional Hospital. He reconfirms the levels of blockages and recommends I be immediately scheduled for a quadruple bypass.

_____

10. Morbidity rate is the percentage of people who have complications from a medical condition or after a procedure or treatment.

He has just upped my game from a triple bypass to a quad. I wasn't happy about the promotion. Apparently, on detailed examination of the angiogram, there was another artery around the back that also presented a blockage. Somewhere in the discussion, he mentions the word, "cabbage."

I hold a hand up. "Cabbage?"

He smiles. "Cabbage is for 'coronary artery bypass grafting' or 'CABG.'"[11]

"Oh!" I'm glad I learned that short hand, because it's commonly used by the OR prep team and the nursing staff in the Cardiac Care Unit. This way, I didn't have to live in wonder at the ubiquitous acronym.

Dr. S explains the coronary artery bypass process in detail, including where in the leg and chest an artery and veins would be harvested as replacements for the sections of artery that needed replacing.

I remember my wife and I were intensely attentive to this discussion, but now it seems to have flown into history. For me at least, I had the mental distraction of what these intrusions might feel like. I tried not to imagine the instrument that was going to split my breastbone.

When asked what our immediate schedule was like, we realize that we needed little time to prepare and had

---

11. A surgical procedure performed to shunt blood around a narrowing or blockage in one or more of the coronary arteries of the heart that usually involves grafting one end of a segment of vein or artery removed from another part of the body into the aorta and the other end of the segment into the coronary artery beyond the obstructed area to allow for increased blood flow.

few reasons to put off the eventual procedure. But I also wanted to get my 69th birthday on September 1st behind me before the surgery. Therefore, we were scheduled for September 5th. Only four and a half months after that initial annual checkup with my nurse practitioner, I'm talking to a cardiac surgeon about a very serious, but routine, procedure.

He says I would probably not be a candidate for the "off pump" technique he's been investigating, where the heart is not disengaged from its pumping duties. Studies reveal that this method is beginning to show inferior results.

Mine will be a typical bypass procedure, where the heart's duties are taken over by a pump, its beating is stopped, and the new segments of arterial and venous tissue are replaced.

I feel a little better about being offered the trusted offline version. Tried and true is good. He tells us not to worry, that over 800,000 of these operations are done worldwide each year.

I think of the people I know who are in the "zipper club," and I still think he might be off by an extra zero. It seems incredible that there are 800,000 of these operations done annually.

He anticipates a morbidity rate of about 2%. I nod and ask if that is 2% for the general population or for me. That is for me: my age, my background, my health issues (there are few), my weight, my cholesterol levels, my genetics, etc. The answer is a little chilling—that 2% accounts for my individual profile. Yes, there's

a 98% chance of survival, leaving a 2% chance of... not surviving.

To me, 2% seems like a big number. In 1980, there was only a 5% chance of a baby being premature. My daughter elected to join that 5% club. Thanks to all the incredible medical help at the time, she's now a licensed mental health counselor. But 2% of that very large number, 800,000, is a lot of not-so-positive outcomes. A quick mental operation obliterates a few seconds of reassurances as I come up with 16,000 unsuccessful outcomes. (I don't remember if that's mortalities or cases that required additional interventions.) Then there's the 98%; a very large number of people survive bypass surgeries and go on to live productive extra years they would not otherwise have had.

The interval from August 21st to September 5th is a little over two weeks and gives me plenty of time for preparation. I haven't any way to do a survey to see if this is common, but the gap in that 98% success rate rattled me. I feel the looming approach of September 5th as an ominous shadow.

How often do we face mortality? We take ridiculous risks in traffic weekly. If the driver behind, in front or beside us does something stupid at the same time we do, either one of us could spin out into a utility pole, semi-truck or other obstacle. Thousands of our present-day youth do as I did in my time and face deployment to

the world's worst neighborhoods. My trip to Southeast Asia in 1969 was an experience shared with friends in uniforms, yet most of us never discussed any misgivings about coming back in a box.

Somewhere between that fuzzy general deployment uncertainty and a professionally stated 2% chance of having my last meal on September 4th, I was nervous.

Some minor preparation was definitely called for. In our mid- to late-60s, my wife and I had not completed a living will, so we opted to complete a document called "Five Wishes." It covers the basic choices and conditions where you would not want to have extraordinary, or any extra, efforts made to keep you alive if you have no expectation of coming out of a coma. There are a few other areas to be filled out, but the repetition in the questioning takes ambiguity out of the document. I'd recommend it.

I also finished a different document as a sort of memoir, outlining the high and low points of my childhood that I would want to share with my daughters.

As for other arrangements, I decided what to do with any unsold copies of my books. I'm also a multiplayer gamer. I share a long-term strategy game with about 70 to 80 other players. If my account is unprotected over a long, drowsy recovery period, I'd lose a lot of invested time and resources. Trivial, I know, but I arranged for another player to take over the account for a few days.

Doing these minor tasks helped me get over the jitters. Were my jitters justified? Maybe not. I did have excellent outcomes. But I'm getting ahead of myself.

Chapter 6

Surgery

Wednesday, September 5th

MORNING WEIGHT, 222.4 LBS. I always check.

We arrive in the predawn coolness and make our way up to Regional Hospital's surgical waiting room. The desk attendant checks her records and notes I am a bypass patient. She is the first of seventeen people who will ask me today to recite my full name and date of birth.

She also tells my wife where to expect me to be after surgery, when that might be, and to call her (by name, if necessary) if she needs *anything*. It is going to be 4 to 6 hours of anxious waiting for my wife and later my daughter. I'm comforted that the staff showed this compassionate concern for my next of kin.

"Any questions?" she asks.

Yes, thousands... But nothing seems to bubble into sound.

We are escorted through a working pre-op ward for catheterizations, stents and many of the other surgical procedures regularly done at Regional Hospital. I scan left and right into darkened, curtain-lined areas with patients looking either apprehensive, sedated or asleep.

Soon, soon. I'm no longer thinking about the 2%. I want this over, and I have a 98% chance of waking up in 4 to 6 hours!

We meet a couple of surgery prep specialists who get me changed into another rear-access gown. They shaved me in almost all the right places. (Unfortunately, my Mediterranean heritage makes me a hairy guy. My wife jokingly asks if they can do my back as well.) Next, they connect me to an electrocardiogram harness that will be with me for the next four days. I've already had a catheter recently inserted into my right wrist's artery, so they insert an IV connection into my left wrist's artery and prepare the saline drip.

The initial team is joined by others specific to the cardio bypass. I am shaved from just below the clavicles to just above my navel; a strip about nipple-to-nipple wide.

A blood oxygen/heart-rate monitor lead is attached to my left middle finger. I don't remember much beyond this. Someone very likely told me that I'd begin to feel

drowsy. I honestly cannot remember. I say goodbye to my wife at 7:15 a.m. and count down from 100 to about 93.

In the waiting room, my wife is joined by my daughter, who will be there for company and support until she needs to leave to pick up my grandson from school. It's going to be a long day for everyone. Help each other out!

For the next several hours, many talented and well-trained technicians and professionals have my life and, quite literally, my heart in their hands. I don't recommend looking up the procedure on YouTube. The images are going to be something you don't want to take with you into pre-op. And besides, techniques vary from medical center to medical center, and they are improving all the time, but the basics are still there. My chest will be opened via an incision down the center of my sternum and stretched apart wide enough for hands to manipulate my heart. Veins and an artery will be harvested from elsewhere to replace the damaged sections of the arteries serving my heart muscle.

The surgeon's notes indicate the first cut was made at 8:24 a.m.

Chapter 7

Waking Up and Beating the 2%

I'M OUT OF SURGERY BY ABOUT 1:00 P.M. and am moved to the room I'll be in until discharge. Not all surgical centers offer this, but my surgeon demands it for his patients. And this is important. It means I'll be seen and supported by the same team of nurses and techs, with decreasing levels of personal support as my condition improves over the next several days. I will not be moved from a cardiac intensive care unit to some other recovery area with different staff.

My support team (my wife and daughter) is told I'll need about an hour for the team to prepare me and the room. The effects of anesthesia fade. Waking up is surreal. Faces crowd close to me on the left and right. It seems dark, or at least blurry.

My first thought on regaining consciousness is, "I woke up!" My two-percenter fears have been unfounded. My team is there with the Cardiac Surgery

Intensive Care Unit's[12] (CSICU) charge nurse, Tonya, and my day shift head nurse, Helen.

As I drift in and out, they explain to my wife and daughter that I need to be further awake before the breathing tube can be removed. They head off for lunch and mutual support while I float ever closer to reality.

About 2:15 p.m., nurses Tonya and Helen are hovering angelically overhead. They tell me they are ready to remove the breathing tube. I nod. No vocal response is possible. I remember fullness, but not a choking sensation.

I've seen enough patient intubations in TV scenarios to have hoped to never need one. But the tube was never in when I was at a level of consciousness to be really aware of the thing. They tell me I should prepare for a good cough. One. Two. Three. Cough. *Ouch*! Painful, yes, but immediately, breathing is easier.

Near 5 o'clock that first afternoon, I'm still fading in and out. Voices float in and out of the anesthetic fog. I can't determine direction, but as I regain focus, my wife is on my left. To my right is a very attractive nurse, Helen. She is asking questions like, "Do you know where you are? Do you know your name?" My wife and daughter are both in the room and asking all the questions a concerned spouse and a trained nurse (my daughter has a Bachelor's of Science in Nursing) might think of.

---

12. An intensive care unit specializing in post-operative heart cases.

The rest of the afternoon is hard to remember. I wonder as I'm writing this if it is simply the aftereffects of the anesthesia or if there is a mild memory blocker in the medicinal cocktail administered.

My wife remembers standing by as Nurse Helen monitors my stats and adjusts the bed and connections for comfort. I'm told later that I shamelessly asked Helen for a date. Maybe more than once. She was lovely, and I was glad to be alive, and I don't remember a word of it.

Helen continually checks the readouts and answers all those questions. I'm feeling pretty good to be alive, back in the world and—I'm alive!

As I become more responsive, I'm asked to breathe into an incentive spirometer. I try to breathe slowly but I'm immediately aware of pain in the center of my chest when I take anything more than a shallow breath.

I manage 500 ml. Half a liter. More on this contraption later.

I drift in and out of anesthesia's waning grip as the afternoon passes into night.

It is not anticipated that I will have an appetite, so the food cart rolls by. Wednesday evening's shift change is through the 7 o'clock hour, and night nurse Taylor comes on. I seem to remember a special delivery of applesauce, which I was able to eat but not finish. The room is darkened, and I hope for sleep to come.

My wife is determined to maintain an overnight vigil but is confronted with the reality of a particularly uncomfortable side chair as the only sleeping option beyond the waiting room. It might be okay for casual seating, but it proves useless as a lounger.

My wife ends her long day and goes home around 9 p.m. She's been up with me since 5 a.m. and has dealt with a lot more anxiety than I have.

I'm assigned two nurses for the next 24 hours. I'll be in the same room through discharge, but assignment of nurses diminishes as I improve and my needs become less urgent. At this stage, each dayshift and nightshift nurse has only one other patient.

The first night seems long. Like long nights anywhere, the option of watching a clock is more painful than not watching it. The one mounted high on the wall directly across from me is unavoidable. I note every five minutes' passage, the arm-crushing interruption every quarter-hour of the blood pressure cuff taking its measurement, and every moment when my blood oxygen level monitor beeps.

Adjusting to the automated warning system of the blood-oxygen monitor becomes my job and my entertainment. Breathe too slowly or too shallowly and the blood-oxygen monitor sends out a rapid-fire beep-beep. I increase my breathing accordingly. The beeping stops.

Nurse Taylor reminds me I need to be exercising the incentive spirometer. This is a plastic device that can measure the volume of my lungs as they are being filled from as empty as I can make it to as full as I can get it. It isn't total volume because if you slow down, a plunger that floats on the airflow will fall. The idea is to breathe in at a rate that satisfies a good-better-best scale on one side while trying to maximize the volume number on the other.

Part of the problem is that there is now a hinge in my chest where there used to be solid bone joining the left and right rib cages. Drawing air into my lungs causes that joint to flex. They don't want that joint to flex. They want it to heal. The pain is a useful limiting factor here.

This time, I measure 900 ml, almost double my first post-op attempt. The pain is real, but manageable. One of the lessons here will be to deal with the pain but ask for help if it becomes too much.

Another part of the problem is that post-operative patients are susceptible to pneumonia. The lungs have been manipulated in the surgical process, literally pushed around with fingers. That manipulation stimulates the secretion of fluids. One of my objectives will be to keep working that spirometer every few hours to improve my lung capacity and help reduce the chance of pneumonia.

I try to use the incentive spirometer again in the sleepless wee hours before dawn, when I pull an entire

liter of air. I remember having been told to use it several times an hour, but have only used it three times so far.

Chapter 8

Recovery

I HAD INTENDED, when my temporary incarceration at Regional Hospital inspired this book, to give a blow-by-blow of the recovery process. In hindsight, I realize each of your stories will be different, dependent on your pre-existing conditions and the local standards of care. You will likely find good, competent care whether you are in a local hospital with a cardiac specialist on-call, a veteran's hospital, a regional medical center or a major cardiac research center. The experiences at those different levels will vary. So, I'm going to hit the highlights of my care, which I believe was exceptional.

Know that your circumstances, the operating protocols at different institutions, and the preferences of your surgeon will differ. I offer my experience solely to let you know that if you've voluntarily offered yourself up to surgery before a heart attack, then the recovery process will be much different than if you are delivered to a cardiac intensive care unit in an ambulance or the

back seat of a neighbor's car. If you come in with heart, lung or brain tissue damage or have reduced brain function as a result of your heart attack, your recovery may be much different than mine.

Thursday, September 6ᵗʰ – Day 1

The first day of the rest of my life. I'll call Wednesday, the day of the operation, Day 0, because I was not there for so much of it.

I report little or no sleep the night before. On an ambiguous pain scale from 1 to 10, I report about a 7. There is not much sharp pain, unless I move, but there is a general feeling of abuse around my chest, and the EKG leads are all sore spots on the abused soft tissue of my chest muscles.

As I become more aware, I take stock of the several attachments on my body. I still have the blood-oxygen/heart rate monitor on my left middle finger. Its lead is taped down to a complicated harness of syringes or sampling points connected to that left-wrist IV access point. Those various tubes and wires disappear out of view to my left.

There is a large bandage on my neck, just below the right side of my chin. There's a lead to my carotid artery there. There is another venous connection to my circulatory system near the base of my neck, at the right shoulder. Both of these central lines had sterile dressings and allowed for monitoring and medication administration.

Looking down, there is a two-inch-wide bandage holding things in above the wound. My new zipper... I've become a member of the Zipper Club—that society of heart surgery survivors that is growing by 800,000 people a year.

The flesh around that bandage is very tender to the touch. I don't poke at it much after the first two attempts. I just don't go there.

To my surprise, there is a harness of chest tubes attached to my abdomen. I later found out these tubes are used to drain fluid and air from inside the chest.

At the base of the long centerline bandage, two smaller tubes exit my body just above the diaphragm and are harnessed to another, half-inch diameter tube running off to the right over the side of the bed. Thin red fluid collects in the low points then siphons off to a collector at my bedside.

There is yet another tube. I was not aware of its insertion at pre-op, for which I am eternally grateful. A urinary catheter is attached and doing its job, as I should not move from my flat-on-my-back position for a while. The bed can be adjusted to some degree, back up or knees raised. But I don't move.

On my right arm, a blood pressure cuff, installed for the duration, powers up every fifteen minutes. It crushes the life out of my right bicep and slowly takes its measure of systolic[13] and diastolic[14] blood pressure as it relaxes.

---

13. The measure of blood pressure when the heart is contracting and pumping blood from its chambers into the arteries.

14. The measure of blood pressure when the heart is filling.

My wife and nurses make their visits to my bedside, and I realize I am in a total care situation. I don't move. I don't need to move, and I don't want to move.

Any attempt at movement is curtailed by an oxygen tube running across my nostrils and draped over each ear. It is flexible, but is attached over my head to a technically advanced wall that has more attachments and dials than I can imagine or understand.

One of the things I appreciate about the care at Regional is that I went straight from the OR to the CSICU. I didn't have to go to a line-up of post-surgical beds to wait for the dissipation of anesthesia. I was taken from surgery straight to the room I'd be in until I was discharged. From what I learn later, this isn't a common practice at all hospitals, where you may be moved multiple times during your stay.

By 10:00 a.m., I'm rousted out of bed for the first time. The not-quite-useful recliner has been moved into position, and I am out of bed, sitting erect. They have given me a stuffed gray teddy bear that I am to hug in case of an oncoming cough.

I'm told there were formerly just pillows, but now there is the bear. His name is Sir Cough-a-lot. Without fail, different members of the staff tell me the bear will be my friend. However, this is not a soft bear. I wondered a few days later if it was a low-bid response to a request for quotes and as a result was not nearly as soft

as the specifications intended. It is a fuzzy, unyielding bear, not soft.

Applying any pressure at all to the stack of tubing and wires taped over the surgical wound or any of the leads applied the previous morning is excruciating. This bear is not *my* friend.

After my third or fourth refusal in two days to use the bear, I'm provided with a pillow.

But back to my first out-of-bed experience since pre-op... The surgical stack of IV leads is removed from my left arm, which provides a little more mobility.

To my surprise, a physical therapist, Ken, arrives in the room, cheerful and expecting to take me for a walk. I think he's kidding. He's not.

There is a small, toaster-sized monitor that receives the leads from my external pacemaker, blood-oxygen sensor and EKG harness. It is attached to a small basket on the front of a walker. I'm familiar with the make and model, as it's nearly identical to the walker my mom-in-law uses for almost any activity five feet from a handhold.

I'm assisted to a vertical position, and we make it to the doorway of my room. I am at the corner of the nursing command center—a square room surrounded on three sides by glass-fronted patient recovery rooms. This is the Cardiac Surgery Intensive Care Unit.

We progress into the hallway as I take baby steps, amazed both that I can do it and that it takes so much energy. The hallway extends a short distance beyond

the central nurses' station toward a pair of double doors. I begin to slow.

Ken points to a red square on the floor, farther ahead, about twelve feet away. It's hard to miss a twenty-inch square made of red lines about two inches wide. It appears to be the same material as the other floor covering. I couldn't begin to guess its function, but that square is Ken's suggested target for me.

I agree, and we advance toward the red square. This is about as far as I can go, and then we return. I've walked less than 60 feet from my chair. Ken stands ready to catch me as I move back to my room, then promises to be back later.

I'm reinstalled in the bedside chair. Sitting erect will help drain the fluids in my chest cavity toward the chest tubes. The container for that drainage draws a slight vacuum through the collecting liquid, so there is always the soft sound of gurgling in the background. As I become aware of its ubiquitous presence, I hope I'll be able to concentrate on its white noise in order to sleep tonight.

I get a visit from a nutritionist who asks for my preferences for the lunch and evening meals. I make my choices. I'm mindful of the warning from the nursing staff that I may not have an appetite for a few days, but find I'm looking forward to mealtime.

When it arrives, it turns out that I really don't have an appetite. The food is flat (no salt), but I enjoy bland turkey and gravy and try a few of the mixed vegetables.

No Jell-O! I always thought Jell-O came with hospital food. I like Jell-O!

In my spare time, I play with the chest cavity drains. I mentioned these above; they are there to drain the chest cavity of the liquids that build up above the diaphragm. One is positioned to drain the entire area, the other is positioned under a lung. They are about a quarter-inch in diameter and are fed into the half-inch tube that runs off the bed. I play with the thin, blood-red fluid that collects and drain it to the floor as often as I note a collection building up. Napping doesn't come easily.

Thursday evening, Physical Therapist Ken returns. He's a big guy and can handle more of a weight challenge than I present. I'm back on my feet and heading out into the ward again.

To my left, a cautious glance through the curtain of my neighbor's room reveals a man secured to his bed. He appears to be sedated—his mouth is gaping open and his eyes crunched shut in apparent pain. I feel lucky. My surgery was elective. I don't have a nearly dead or damaged mass of heart tissue sending out "please God, come get me" signals.

As we progress, I steal a quick look into the next room. I note a family quietly whispering over the body of an unmoving patient.

We get to the morning's marker and Ken asks if I can do more. It's been easier than earlier, and I'm not too winded. None of the monitors are complaining. I nod, and he taps the automatic door operator. I say, "Beyond Red Square and onward to Siberia." He doesn't seem to get the joke.

There is an intersection of hallways several feet ahead. We turn right and, perhaps 80 feet farther, turn right again through another automated door and back into the CSICU.

If I wanted to, I could have glanced into more of my fellow patients' spaces through open doors or partially opened windows. I don't, I'm satisfied to be up and moving. We break no speed records returning to my room.

My equipment and I are reinstalled into the bed as my exercise is over for the day. Dinner comes, and my wife shares my no-salt heart-healthy offering.

My wife and daughter are here for company, and I'm glad for it. We are told that the little black thing on an opposite wall's cabinet is a TV. *That* is a TV? We share a private joke. Apparently, Regional Hospital's maternity rooms have been fitted with widescreen TVs and electronic whiteboards that display who your assigned nurses are, as well as your most recent vitals. Not here, not yet. My home computer has a larger monitor. But we end up watching the thing until the end of visiting hours.

We watch the opening round of the BMW Championship. It's also the final selection round for

the PGA championship and an important contest for the final selection for the Ryder Cup. It's a big-deal golf contest and one of my long-time favorites is holding his own against a much younger crowd.

Near the end of Day 1, the insulin drip is removed from the IV. The night approaches. Nurse Taylor is back on duty and tells me I should sleep better the second night. The first is usually a hard night. I tell her that even if I begin to drop into sleep, the quarter-hour gripping squeeze of the blood pressure cuff would make it impossible to get any genuine rest. She adjusts its reporting criteria, and I can expect only half-hour interruptions.

Thursday fades very slowly into Friday. I seem to be aware of almost every five-minute interval throughout the night. Each pressurization of the blood pressure cuff occurs about 2 minutes after the hour and half-hour. I don't know if the clock or the equipment is keeping accurate time, but at least they are consistently off.

Taylor quietly comes in and out throughout the night, hoping not to wake me, but ..•sigh••. I'm awake. Glad for the interaction.

The second night goes much as the first. I note the passage of time in five-minute segments, fail to get any meaningful rest and, if sleep does come, the blood pressure cuff cuts it short.

I'm tired, but then nothing is expected of me again today. No sprints, no lifting, little movement.

Friday, September 7th – Day 2

Dr. S arrives at 6:15 a.m. We discuss my progress. He says I'm doing well. I complain about the bear. He looks at the collection equipment for the chest tubes and regrets to tell me that the rate of drainage is still too high. He would have liked to have removed it, but not today. All else appears to be progressing well, he reports. He says the chest tubes will probably be removed the next day. I'm given the hopeful news that I may be released on Sunday, if I keep progressing on schedule.

Friday is essentially another Thursday, except that the accumulated loss of sleep, from two restless nights here at Casa Regional and the night of anticipation, has tired me out. My wife tells me I was grumpier Friday.

Whatever pain medication regime I'm on, it is working. On that 1–10 pain scale, I report a 1 or 2. It's essentially negligible, unless I move. I try not to move as I have good pain avoidance reflexes.

I am supposed to grip the bear to my chest and lock my arms together in order to move. I have no use for the Bear from Hell. I have asked for a spare pillow to hug if I have an impending cough. In order to move, I was supposed to hug Sir Cough-a-lot; instead, I use the pillow.

I've learned to lock my fingers together under my gut, tuck my elbows into my side and move as a tight-muscled solid form. Actually, *to be moved* as a tight-muscled solid form. Any movement into and out of the bed or the chair is assisted by the nurses on duty. I'm not trusted to stand alone.

All this is good. I shouldn't be trusted to stand alone. Blood oxygen can fluctuate rapidly. I can't imagine the grief and suffering I would experience if I was to fall.

My physical therapist, Ken, returns to find me too tired (read: exhausted), and I ask for nap time. This happens, and I get a 2-hour nap Friday afternoon. Sweet relief! I sleep through at least three or four of the blood pressure tests.

By afternoon, I'm refreshed and ready to take on... more rest. I do get into the chair and enjoy several hours of golf, watching the BMW Championship.

Friday afternoon, I meet another of the physical therapy staff. I never catch her name because her name tag seems to be velcroed into a permanent reverse position.

I'm anxious for a walk, but we don't even make it to Red Square. We do two loops around the nurses' station and are back in the room much too soon. She indicates she doesn't like to leave the CSICU because of the increased germ hazard. Hmm, apparently it's dangerous in Siberia or she is behind schedule and needs to move on.

Between the timely visits of the day nurse, Kathy, my wife and I watch another day of the BMW Championship on the cabinet-top TV. We pick at the dinner that has been provided. We find it's not only my surgically impacted palette that finds it hard to stomach. It just isn't very good. I'm told I can expect to lose several pounds because of loss of appetite. I

don't know if that stuff was ever palatable. It's a quiet evening, and I hope for sleep.

At shift change, I meet a new night nurse, Kaitlyn. I find there is a qualitative difference in the individual application of nursing care. From personality to attentiveness, I'm appreciating the difference. When I mention I was disappointed by the truncated afternoon walk, she offers a second hike after she completes her change-of-shift duties. Things were slow initially on that shift, so she came right back.

Our excursion goes far beyond Red Square and out to the second crossing hall. I can feel my increase in strength and stamina. True, I have an elevated heart rate, but my only slightly reduced oxygen levels and rapid heart rate recovery are good signs of improvement. Kaitlyn reports this to me in those quantitative terms, which the physical therapists had not done.

Saturday, September 8th – Day 3

I'm awake on Saturday morning when Dr. S comes in at 6:30. I've *been* awake for quite a while. I think there was an unaccounted-for period between 2:45 and 4:02 a.m. when I was asleep, but the blood pressure cuff got me just after 4 o'clock.

He's checked the accumulating data in my file. I appear to be progressing well. He inspects the drainage from the chest tubes, and I'm a "go" for their removal and a probable release on Sunday!

Kaitlyn and Dr. S make the preparations for the chest tube removal with remarkably tender care. My skin in this area is still over-sensitive, and I appreciate the slow removal of the adhesive bandages and other connections. The chest tubes come out with a lot less discomfort than I'd been anticipating. The oxygen tubes are gone, and I'm aware the slow flow of dry gas has dried out the first half-inch of my nasal passages.

I'm feeling a lot more chipper on Day 3, and my wife arrives just in time for breakfast at 9 a.m. I don't know the reason, but meals have consistently been arriving about two hours later than I would have eaten them on the outside. The eggs are bland, with no salt. The toast is a hard triangle of crisp bread that actually clinks when you tap it on the plate. I eat a little of the grits. It's hard to screw up grits.

No problem… No reason to complain to the staff. I truly do not have an appetite. I'm reminded that this is common after major surgery.

Not only are the chest tubes removed today, but I also lose the arterial connection to my carotids and the central white bandage that has been a stark exclamation point on my chest. I find myself staring down at the scar. It's reasonably straight with purplish knots at irregular intervals. There are residual blood stains in the flexible surgical glue that is holding my chest together.

That evening, I ask Kaitlyn what kind of binder has been used on the breastbone beneath the hot pink scar

running down my centerline. I've been imagining some industrial strength glue, like small single-use tubes of Liquid Nails. (Liquid Bone?) I wonder what level of exertion or flexing my breastbone can take so soon after surgery. Using the incentive spirometer often hits a limit where the centerline of my chest shouts "Stop!" She begins to explain, then pauses. She'll try to come back with an explanatory picture after she checks on her other patient.

Returning, she provides a sketch showing a human rib cage with wire ties running between the ribs and around the sternum, then twisted tight to maintain the contact of bone on bone. Each opening has its own wire. I note that they haven't opened the entire rib cage, only about the upper two-thirds according to the picture. I now have a visual image of the zipper that's been installed in my chest.

I also see two wires inserted below that section. She explains these are the leads to the external pacemaker. I barely remember mention of a pacemaker from my foggy state on Day 1. She checks, finds some of the pacemaker equipment still in place, and removes it.

After that, we take one more promenade around the hallway. This is a bonus for me. It has been a busy day on the ward. Quite a few new neighbors fill the rooms around the CSICU. This has meant not only a number of discharges earlier in the day but more new patients coming in. Although I was meant to be only one of two patients for Kaitlyn, she has two new patients now, one of whom is in great need.

I don't begrudge that. I'm glad I walked into the hospital on my own—that I'm not suffering from heart tissue or brain damage from a heart attack. Those cases looked to be in considerably worse shape.

Saturday night's only bad moments come from the very disappointing performance of my college football team. Once a national champion, we're now playing an early season B-team, and we barely pulled out a win after posting a game with only a few positive yards rushing and not many more in the air.

You can't have everything, right?

Sunday, September 9th – Day 4 (Homecoming)

It's Sunday. I've gotten used to Dr. S arriving before 6:30 a.m. However, today he arrives after 7:30. It is a Sunday though, so no problem.

He checks the wound area and the sutures around the chest tube points. He's checked my charts, and I'm good to go home.

Remember that I had surgery on Wednesday? It seems incomprehensible that I'm going home today. Really? But I feel good. Sure, on Day 4, my stamina is pitiful and energy levels are never high, but I've been making good progress on the incentive spirometer and can pull 2,250 ml. Up from 500 ml on Day 1!

I ask if my last connection to the medico-electronic world, the EKG leads, can be removed, and they are.

I'm writing this section eight days after that Sunday, and the places those leads were attached are the sorest places remaining other than the scar itself.

There has to be a thinner, just as good, disposable lead out there. Regional Hospital has such a tremendous investment in the latest technology. How much can a better EKG lead cost?

By noon, I am wheeled down to Regional Hospital's entrance for a transition to recovery life at home. I've been given three simple rules:

- Don't lift your hands above your head.
- Don't lift more than 10 lbs.
- Don't drive for a month.

I'm also to ask for help getting into and out of bed.

When some home health physical therapists come to the house later, I'm also advised that my hands should not go behind my back. This makes putting on even a light, cotton button-down shirt impossible without help.

I settle into my new parking spot for the next month: my easy chair. It's not a power lift chair or even a power chair. It's an older La-Z-Boy with a hand-cranked lever on the right. That lever needs more than 10 lbs of torque to fully engage the leg lift. Since my legs should be elevated to assist in the elimination of fluids stored in my lower legs, more care is to be required of my ever-supportive wife just to get my legs elevated.

Bear in mind, these are my personal experiences. Every patient will have a different discharge condition and different support team available to assist. If I had not had a good support team, I might well have been discharged from the CSICU to a recovery unit in the hospital or a rehab center. If I had less insurance coverage, I might have investigated some other options. For instance, I could have requested admission to the new Veterans Administration facility. The regional VA hospital happens to be in my hometown and would have been convenient if I hadn't misplaced my VA medical ID card.

I am fortunate enough to have been sent home to a secure environment where most of my needs could be met by my wife. Fortunately, home nursing and physical therapy care services were offered, and we accepted. This was set up in advance and we had our first nursing visit on my second day home.

Monday, September 10th – Day 5

I wake after first light, around 7 a.m. Heart rate monitoring has become a daily part of my statistics ritual.

My first day after surgery, I played games with the blood-oxygen/heart rate monitor to keep its alarm from sounding. Now, five days later, I set my Apple Watch to monitor my heart rate. It won't do BP or temperature. The Apple Watch is an exercise watch, not a health monitor.

My morning weight of 222.4 lbs was very close to my check-in weight prior to surgery.

This first morning at home I enjoy eating real food.

One of our first orders of business is finding a wedge pillow to help with sleep comfort. We order, rush delivery, a foam wedge pillow from Amazon to mimic the elevated bed in the hospital and to make it more likely I will remain asleep on my back.

Tuesday, September 11th – Day 6

Amazon got our order Monday morning, and we received the pillow Tuesday afternoon. Isn't the 21st century grand?

The wedge pillow allows a slight elevation of the head. It's helpful to stay on my back because, for now, moving to either side puts stresses on that wire-stitched sternal joint. I don't want that. I actually find that moving to sleep on either side is about a 3 or 4 on the pain scale, so I stay on my back for about a week.

One day back and I'm feeling pretty good. Yes, it hurts to move suddenly. It hurts to push or pull. Obeying guidance to not put my arms over my head means my wardrobe is limited. I have an extended collection of t-shirts from simple undergarments to concert shirts, location shirts, and tees of all descriptions. I can't wear any of them.

I have maybe eight to ten lightweight, summer, button-down, cotton shirts. These are the go-to shirts of the day and for the next few weeks. I can put them on

without lifting my arms over my head, and they can be left partially unbuttoned so as to not lay on top of the still very sensitive wound area. For you guys with fur on your chest, you will be growing a bristle brush on the skin surrounding that wound.

Today, I receive my first visits from home health and home physical therapy. Nursing care goes over the obvious medical history and sets up a schedule of three visits next week, two the following, and then one a week until otherwise advised. Although I feel physically in good shape after the surgery, there is still the potential for pneumonia, infection and secondary injury to the surgical sites.

The physical therapist shows up two hours later. In that first session, we review my baseline heartrate and my potential exercise regimen. Her routine includes stamina and strength testing.

In retrospect, I'm a little disappointed that neither the nurse nor the PT tech is interested in the breathing routine recommended by the hospital to keep my lungs free of water, to repair stressed alveoli, and to keep me alive as long as other things don't go wrong. Today's best reading on the incentive spirometer, a Voldyne 5000, is 2,250 ml.

Thursday, September 12th – Day 8

I've been out of the hospital for four days and post-op for eight days. I feel pretty good until I walk farther than the length of the hallway. I get up almost too often

to relieve my bladder, which is receiving the desired effects of the diuretic. This is a good thing. Not only is the short trip down the hall necessary from the bladder's point of view, but it's a short and often-repeated work-out.

Exercise and recovery are the mode for the next several weeks. Physical therapy and nursing are provided by a home health service at the Memorial Hospital. We heard, even in Regional Hospital, that Memorial's post-operative home health services were better. I won't judge since I haven't been through both.

The exercise routines are simple and doable, and will escalate in intensity as I am able. Yesterday, the PT tech and I walked around the back of the house to the driveway. He asked if I was doing okay. I said, "Let's go get the mail, as long as you're here to catch me."

He didn't need to catch me. I made it down the slope of the drive to the mailbox, got the mail and we returned. My heart rate was humming at about 112 beats per minute (bpm) but, to our mutual satisfaction, quickly settled down to the mid-80s.

My recovery isn't expected to be horrendously long. My physical therapist's assigned goal for me is to add another driveway each day. I'll walk my neighborhood and simply add one more driveway each time.

In one direction, the return trip is all uphill. So I resolve to go in the other direction. In this neighborhood, each additional mailbox is another 120 feet or so. After dinner today, my wife and I added one more mailbox.

Physical therapy plans to be back twice a week for the next two weeks, then for a final visit in the third, ending much sooner than we'd thought. I am hoping the prognosis is that good. I still won't be able to drive for thirty days after surgery, but I can live with that.

I am abundantly aware that I have a new lease on my natural life span if I correct the dietary and sedentary abuses I've been subjecting my heart and body to for the past three decades.

At 30, my waist was 30″. At 50, it was 38″, and it stayed there for almost two decades. So, assuming I avoid getting cancer and don't step in front of a bus, I might make it several years, maybe a couple of decades, beyond the lifetimes of my parents.

I'll have to hope my memory lasts at least as long as all those other systems.

The biggest issues of the first few days back from my luxury stay at Regional Hospital are simple things: getting into and out of bed. This will require help from my wife for a few more days at least. Until the soreness at the sternum subsides, I still can't sleep on my side. So, chair-bound by day and flat on my back by night, my buttocks and back get sore. And so do my shoulders, from lack of flexing. The directives remain: no weight over 10 lbs, get assistance in chair and bed maneuvers, and continue to work out my lungs on the incentive spirometer.

Sunday, September 15th – Day 11

I get up and around much more easily. I no longer require assistance getting into and out of bed. I confirmed this with my physical therapist, showing him how I do the drop-and-flop technique I was taught at the hospital. With a nurse's assistance, I'd tuck at the waist and, with bent knees, would fall onto the bed on my side while the nurse lifted my legs.

At home, I learned to convert that falling motion into a roll that left me on my back. During this maneuver, I keep my core, chest and arms rigid. But it works pretty well and, with practice, I end up with my head on the pillow.

I'm not sure my wife would have given up trying to be there each time unless the physical therapist had okayed it.

Getting up is another matter. I use a mixed menu of tightening core muscles and extending my legs into space to counterbalance my body. As my weight shifts outward and I begin to roll to the side, I flex my supporting arm at the elbow, levering my body almost upright. If there's someone handy to gently pull on the free arm, that's even better.

I learned that technique one night in a hurry while responding to a cramp in my calf muscle. Remember those muscle cramps from the beginning of this odyssey? They're still here.

Because the orders that limit movement are designed to keep me from exerting stresses on my rib cage, the

primary restrictions limit my ability to lift the leg support on my easy chair. I spend most of my day there and, about half of that time, my legs should be up to assist the diuretics in de-watering. This means another demand on my very busy wife—lifting my legs up.

I'm not sure how much longer I will have to be on the Spironolactone, but the low-potassium cramps still occur. I had one last night and a doozy this morning just before breakfast that persisted (or tried to) for over four minutes.

My weight is dropping significantly. A morning weight of 216.4 lbs seemed like an impossible dream last year when I was trying not to go over 235. Getting above 235 lbs was going to require giving up entirely on a waist size of 38 and financing a wardrobe in the 40 line. It was simply getting too uncomfortable to fasten that top button on too many of my pairs of pants. For years, 235 lbs had been my upper winter limit and, after some struggle, I usually got down to 230 lbs for summer. This is me struggling with a need to eat, maintaining poor road food habits, and losing those inner debates on whether to satisfy a need to hit an extra drive-thru more than three or four times a week.

My wife and daughter cook good, low-fat, low-carbohydrate foods for our weekly (or more often) family meals. If those were all I ate, I might not be here writing this. I tried once to see a shrink about the issue, to find out the driving forces behind that need to satisfy cravings with food. That didn't go well. Sure, I had a crappy childhood, but so what? Lots of us did. The struggle

will be to recognize the driving urge when it's driving. Driving me into the drive-thru lane… Driving me into the door of the convenience store when I only needed gas… Driving me along the road to the *next* coronary event…

Regardless of the shrink's admonitions and advice, I have an oral fixation that got resolved too often with various gas station food: cookies, peanut-butter candy bars and 2-for-$2 hot dogs.

I know I'm not alone, or these markets wouldn't be there. A gas station owner told me once that he didn't really make a profit on gas; it's too competitive with the three other guys at the intersection. He made a living selling soft drinks, beer and snacks. He sold only about one bunch of bananas in an entire day, but he required several vendors' visits a week to keep his shelves stocked.

Wednesday, September 18th – Day 14

I'm still in the recovery routine: I've been lifting nothing over 10 lbs, haven't been reaching over my head, and still haven't gotten into my truck.

Getting into and out of bed is something I can do on my own now. I still prefer to sleep on my back, causing the inevitable buzz saw. My wife still prefers to distance herself from the up-close rendition of my snoring. (She sleeps in the guest room.) And I'm still losing weight!

When the PT techs come, they have me stand next to the kitchen sink and do leg lifts to raise my heart rate. The first one that came stopped me at 65 lifts when my breathing became labored. The last one to visit stopped me at 200 and concluded I could be discharged.

My heart rate recovery from staged exercise is good. I can go from 110 bpm to 85 in just a minute or two. My stamina is increasing too. On my walks, I'm not adding much distance, but my pace has gone up. I still try to keep my bpm under 110, but this can usually be accomplished by remembering to breathe deeply.

Usually, when we walk, we don't think about consciously breathing deeper. Our bodies respond automatically via the autonomous nervous system that controls that stuff. I find I need to make that effort when out walking to keep from getting too light on my feet.

So, this is still very much a goal: more walking, adding a bit more each day. It's late September here in North Florida and today, for instance, we're looking at a heat index of over 100°F. At this stage in recovery, battling inclement elements isn't on the menu. I try to get out and walk before 9:00 a.m. or wait until dusk.

Whatever your conditions as you face your recovery routine, don't push your luck—no snow, no icy ground, no rain, mud or poor visibility. Think of yourself as an invalid. If you have to do laps in your house, do so. If you can't get away from poor weather, get driven to a mall or even a grocery store to walk. Walking is going to become your friend.

Sleeping has gotten easier. Tonight, I will try to sleep normally in bed, without the wedge pillow providing additional elevation. I've found that lately, I end up sliding down and curling (yes, curling!) into a modified fetal position.

I'm not sure if it's medically advisable, but I can get temporary relief by sleeping for short periods on my left or right side. I've had a small pillow at my side to provide some support for a slight variation of flat on my back. I find that, now, I can hug that pillow, giving some support to my arms as I sleep on one side or the other.

I make several trips to the head each night as I pay homage to the diuretics. I usually have several mouthfuls of water before heading back to sleep. Water in, water out. The need to purge from the diuretics must be maintained by the need to remain hydrated. It's a yin-yang, Mr. Miyagi, wax on/wax off kind of thing. Remember, abstaining from that restorative drink of water doesn't mean you won't be up again in two hours. Get used to it.

Two weeks after the surgery, I'm feeling stronger and aware that many who go through this post-op experience have a tendency to fall into depression. Yes, movement and activity and all the things I was doing prior to two weeks ago are either on hold or are more limited. I have the support of an attentive wife and daughter. I'm reading more and watching interesting television shows. I am *not* becoming addicted to the drivel shoveled up

for daytime broadcast television. (Sorry, you might like fake judges and who's-your-daddy shows…)

My point is, I'm doing my level best to keep my mind active and stimulated. Writing this book is helping, by the way.

I realize I am the result of all-American advertising that has consistently advised me to get the next incarnation of America's best hamburger or limitless pasta night or all-you-can eat Americana buffets or happy-hour milkshakes.

I watched. I drove in. I ate. I became obese. I could have died.

Tuesday, September 24th – Day 20 (Follow-Up)

The follow-up appointment with Dr. P is enlightening. Another EKG and blood pressure test are taken prior to the interview. I ask about the prognosis for continued edema with the correction of blood flow to the heart. This leads to an additional discussion of the initial suggestion of congestive heart failure.

Dr. P said I probably did not have congestive heart failure since my heart tissues did not appear to have suffered any damage. He assures me the pedal edema should clear up. Cognitively, I'm back to asking what the connection is between heart disease and edema.

I tell him I still have swelling in my ankles. He nods. "Yes, but you had a vein removed and blood and fluids

are still trying to figure out alternate routes back to the heart."

A quick check confirms there is still some swelling in the right leg, which donated the veins for the bypass, but not so much in the left leg. There's very little sign of swelling on the left ankle. Hmmm...

So, the pedal edema was caused by the weakened heart tissue not being able to maintain the pressure required to pump blood back up the venous system to the heart. I do not appear to have pulmonary edema, which is fluid buildup in the chest cavity.

In fact, he drops the prescription to the Spironolactone, the diuretic with its additional complication of leg cramps. There's no need to taper off. So, hopefully, I've taken the last of those and will no longer have any more 3:00 a.m. cramping events.

Monday, October 8th – Day 34

All things must come to an end. Today, I see my cardiac surgeon for the post-op appointment. Yesterday, I attended my first fitness session at the Wellness Center sponsored by Regional Hospital. Between these two milestones, my family and the rest of Tallahassee prepared for the arrival of Hurricane Michael. I mention this only because those preparations tested the limits of the post-op directive to avoid lifting any more than 10 lbs.

The morning session at the Wellness Center consisted of lower body workouts on an elliptical bike, a

treadmill and a recumbent bike. At each new machine, my blood oxygen, blood pressure and heart rate were evaluated.

I managed pretty well with these, but the talk of the morning was the impending arrival of Hurricane Michael. It was expected to hit my section of the Gulf coast in two days. I was given a copy of my heart's performance readings on the three machines to take to my appointment later with Dr. S.

The appointment with my surgeon had been on my mind for several days, for less than obvious reasons. It had been postponed from the prior Tuesday, and I was anxious about the removal of two stitches that remained around the two incisions for the chest tubes. The small tails of these stitches looked as if the material they were made of was cotton with tiny fibrous filaments. I was concerned the fibrous material of the thread might become one with my skin.

Dr. S arrives and immediately asks to see the surgical site, my new zipper scar. It looks pretty good to me, and he agrees. Most of the dark areas I had seen in the early weeks were due to residual glue that has been slowly eroding in the shower over the past month. The scar is a light pink line running almost straight down the center of my chest. The two chest tube incisions a half-inch lower have their little stitch tails dangling below.

My doctor reaches for a small pair of scissors in his pocket, snips one of the loops, and pulls on the knotted end. To my great relief, the thread slides right out. The only thing I feel is a slight tugging sensation on the skin. Whew! The second stitch comes out as smoothly as the first. Double whew! All that anxiety for nothing. It turns out, the stitches are made of nylon and they weren't permanently bonding with my flesh.

At the conclusion of the visit, I'm cleared to drive again and to slowly start lifting heavier weights than the post-op 10-pound limit. That's good because preparation for Hurricane Michael is a necessity. Some of the plants I remove from the deck later weigh close to 40 lbs. My generator is on wheels, but it weighs in at over 100 lbs.

There were no adverse effects from this extra effort, but the labor of clearing the deck of movable objects reminds me that the clearance to drive and slowly increase activity is not carte blanche to do whatever I feel like doing. It wears me out. I go back to that earlier admonition from the cardiologist: slow and steady progress. Don't push it.

Chapter 9

Observations

THE DAY BEFORE THE VISIT to Dr. P, another complication did arise. Lower back pain. I first felt it as kidney pain. A quick check of the side effects of my medications provided no clues as to a possible connection. No chair, couch or stool provided any relief. By mid-afternoon, I resorted to my bed, hoping that lying down would help. The familiar twinge of muscle pull as I got back into bed provided the clue.

My technique for getting into and out of bed required stiffening my core muscles and taking the strain of getting vertical or horizontal on the lower back muscles, probably the external obliques. I spent that afternoon, evening and night on my back in bed. By dawn, I could walk with only vestigial pain in that muscle group. To protect those muscles from further damage, I switched which side of the bed I slept on. This exercised the other side of my back when I had to get up. Explaining all this

to Dr. P got me a scrip for Flexeril, a muscle relaxer, in case the pain persisted.

Apparently, I'm doing fine. The prognosis is for a slow and gradual recovery. Reader, listen to the emphasis on *slow and gradual*. Things are still going to be sore, but you are improving at this point. If for any reason, something does not seem right, do not hesitate to call your physician.

There is remaining soreness in my chest from tissue trauma when the two sides of my chest were levered open for the surgery. Remember that they make one vertical incision in the chest down the middle? They stretch that into a rectangle using retractor clamps. The soft tissues of the chest will continue to feel that abuse for months to come.

I am advised by Dr. P to join a physical therapy group for other post-bypass patients. The next step will be the follow-up appointment with the surgeon, Dr. S.

In the last week, I've taken longer and longer walks each day. As the earlier advice recommended, I added one extra driveway each day.

Movement, stamina and endurance have all increased in small increments. I water the plants in the backyard, and this feels like a victory.

My Apple Watch is an especially useful tool on my walks. After the initial "one more mailbox" phase, I jumped to around the block, then around twice. However, at each corner or the end of each rise, I check my heart rate, let it recover to less than 105 bpm, then continue on.

Several watches and fitness bands are available that will give you this information.

Appetite and Diet

With all that I've been through, obviously I have new inspiration to adopt a heart-healthy diet. I'd advise you too to start listening and paying attention to those guidelines. Just because you are overweight doesn't mean you need to try a fancy boutique diet. Just lower the fat content and eat smaller portions. It might be a good time to ask your cardiologist or cardio-surgeon to recommend a dietitian who isn't driven by a profit motive to get you healthier.

In these first days after surgery I had almost no appetite. Almost a week back from the hospital, I still do not get hungry on time. So far, enough relatives and friends have been generous with meal deliveries that we have a stack of possible meals and leftovers in the fridge. These are working for now, and my wife and daughter, my primary cooks, are well-versed in cooking light.

Personal Care

Upon arriving home from the hospital after my surgery, I'm feeling particularly gross from layers of antiseptic wash still adhering to my skin. A thickening neck beard seems to be coated in the stuff. We shower. No, my wife showers me in our master bath's shower. She is attentive and careful. We are both afraid to touch "the wound." In two days, I'll be patting it down with more pressure

and less trepidation. But for that first shower, we are cautious and careful.

I get into my pajama shorts and am anxious to check for the predicted weight loss. I ate almost nothing between midnight on Tuesday prior to surgery and the very tiny meal I was able to get down Thursday, with only very small meals since then. I am bummed. I weigh in at 225.6 lbs, three more than I weighed on Wednesday morning.

I look down at a distended belly and see signs of the added weight coming from water retention in my bowels and body. The Spironolactone has much more work to do to get rid of my water weight.

Showers should be a two-person event at first. It's good to have an intimate friend there. We happen to have a shower chair because mom-in-law is bathed in our walk-in shower. It's handy for me now. Since it's unlikely you have a hospital-grade shower chair, a plastic lawn chair will do.

You can't shower yourself without disobeying the directives on arm movement. Just trying to do it yourself the first few days will cause you pain. You should not feel pain. If you do, you are stressing the joint in your chest that is held together for now with only glue and wires. Avoid pain.

Discomfort is expected. I'm home on pain medications as needed, but I only take them at bedtime. Still, even with pain meds, you must avoid pain. If you don't want an emergency medical team opening up that zipper again, do not shower by yourself.

Weight Loss

Back in the hospital, when I had no appetite and the sodium-free food was barely palatable, I was told to expect to lose some weight. It seemed like a reasonable expectation. Since coming home, I've also been eating much better food and smaller portions. In the expectation that you might have similar experiences, I'll share my weight loss results.

I've already reported my weight of 222.4 lbs on the morning of surgery and the surprising increase to 225.6 lbs on my return home. The weight did begin to fall off.

Initially, it wasn't obvious, as there were fluids built up in my chest and gut that the Spironolactone was helping with. But the reduced intake in the hospital and eating for a smaller appetite on returning home began to show up in the daily record. I bottomed out in the 212 range and began to regain some weight. This is when the effects of the diuretic finally left my system and I stabilized at about 214 lbs.

From here on, it will be longer walks, more exercise, and vigilant adherence to a healthier diet. I will admit to still jonesing for snack food. Those cravings will have to be re-addressed to healthier alternatives that have been there all along: grapes, apples, bananas, etc.

Sleep

We were told many patients come home to live day and night in their easy chairs. This does not come to pass

for me. My recliner is comfortable enough, and I've fallen asleep in it on more than a few occasions, but I had never spent the night intentionally.

I made it to about 3:00 a.m. before I gave up and we headed for the bedroom. We piled some pillows at the head of the bed and tried to repeat the flip-and-roll procedure the nurses at Regional had used. My wife slept in the guest room with a baby monitor turned on so I could call for assistance getting out of and back into bed.

On my back, I snore loudly and the only position I can sleep in now is on my back. For that reason, she sleeps at a remove in the spare bedroom, where she can attenuate my snoring with the volume control on a baby monitor and still hear me if I needed help.

Sleeping on my side is hard-to-impossible at this early stage. To inhibit the urge to roll on my side, we bought that wedge pillow. It does make it harder, in sleep mode, to roll to one side or the other. Another partial solution is to use one of the frou-frou pillows my wife keeps on the bed as a sort of back rest. With that wedged under one side, I can be at rest in a partially turned position without putting a lot of weight on my shoulder, which then transfers to my chest and hurts.

The simple pressure of a sheet on the tender and abused soft tissues of my chest is irritating and sometimes downright painful. I learn to steeple my hands over my chest, creating a tent pole for the sheet. By the time I move or shift and the sheets settle, I've made

it deeply enough into sleep that I don't wake from the discomfort.

Boredom

Even hurricane coverage isn't enough. I completed a series I'd been watching on Netflix, and I'm finishing some books. It's easy to get a subscription to Audible, which has an incredible variety of books to help make your recovery hours slip by.

You'll end up annoyed that you have to get up again already to service the needs of the diuretics, but at least it's a break in the monotony.

Money Matters

I am fortunate to be a member and beneficiary of one of this country's top ten health maintenance organizations. The quality of HMOs varies widely with total membership, location, competition and other market variables. Mine has a wide and well-funded membership of university, state and local government employees as well as the employees of my home city's three major higher education institutions. This large base provides a significant financial base to fund medical services for its membership.

I am also retired, and the HMO partners with Medicare to further supplement the level of support. If you belong to an HMO and are retired, make sure you can get the complementary coverage. The same would go for any other insurance you might have, as

well as the Veterans Administration. Be sure to check these avenues out if you are planning on an elective procedure.

After a heart attack, you will still need to figure this out, but you won't be as mobile. Getting to the right offices will be difficult for several weeks.

I won't get into the exact specifics of my case, but in round numbers, my surgery alone cost upward of $250,000. The stress test and catheterization added another several thousand dollars. My co-pay for the testing was $40 each, the standard office visit co-pay within my HMO. My co-pay for the surgery was $200. Later, I received a "This is not a Bill" notice from the HMO telling me the other attending professionals had charged another $20,000, paid by them.

So again, I feel very fortunate for my specific circumstances. If I was not covered, I might not have paid for the two testing procedures because of the expense. It could have paid for a decent used car! If I had had any inkling of the cost of the surgery, I would have been devastated by the choice. You can get a loan for a car; you can mortgage a house. But you cannot take out a loan with your body as collateral.

For many, the choice is made for them as they wake up in recovery. They have been delivered to the emergency room in the back of an ambulance and no longer have the option of planning ahead.

It is estimated that over 600,000 Americans per year declare bankruptcy when faced with the enormous financial burden of open-heart surgery. Lost homes,

dissolved marriages, depression and other psychological or physical complications can result from these devastating debts.

I won't get into the political background of why this is so. I'll just mention that for the majority of the developed world, the cost of open-heart surgery is $0.00 or, rather, £0.00, €0.00 or ¥0.00. Some version of national healthcare pays the bill.

But you don't live there, do you? So, see about getting insured. Do whatever you possibly can to acquire insurance. Even the base rate in the U.S., with a $5,000 to $6,000 deductible, is preferable to $250,000 or more of unexpected debt thanks to your heart attack.

This might seem Pollyannaish. How can I be so simple-minded?

There is an option. Stop planning to have your heart attack. Start planning to *not* have a heart attack. All it comes down to is diet and exercise. I'm sure your physician has been harping at you for years to mend your ways. Walking is your friend. It doesn't require a gym membership; it can be done in fair weather or in a mall in inclement weather.

Am I sounding pedantic now? You bet your life I am. As I finish these final thoughts, I'm four and a half weeks out of surgery. I walk over two miles a day. I'm anticipating longer walks when the temperatures in Florida drop below 90°.

As a new member of the Zipper Club, I feel fine. I'm still working up to the simple things, like driving my truck or mowing my own lawn. Those things

will come with time. I'm starting a fitness routine next week at the Wellness Center that will track my increased capabilities.

I'm not writing this book with any interest in making vast sums of money. I simply want others to know what to expect. To possibly keep a few of my readers from being as ignorant as I was going in and to keep a few of you from needing the procedure at all.

My condition, if it had not advanced to the 80% blockage levels in three arteries, might have been mitigated with those two simple changes in lifestyle: diet and exercise. Sorry, but you have to do this yourself.

The alternative, doing nothing, or rather continuing to do what you are doing now, taking your pear-shaped self along the road to cardiac distress, may possibly end with you needing to write your own chapters. Good luck, and I mean that.

Chapter 10

Complications

I HAD THE OPPORTUNITY to sit down with supervising Nurse A the December after my surgery. The nurses under her work long hours bringing their patients back to a level of health that doesn't require intensive care. As I've discussed before, I spent four days under their care.

My journey, I had been told, was a textbook case of how to do it right. But I didn't really know what that meant. I suspected the patients I'd seen in the ward, who laid unmoving for days, had a much harder road to recovery. To complete this story, I felt I needed to find out what happens when a patient doesn't come in through the hospital's front door. What happens when a patient arrives in an ambulance?

To answer this question, I interviewed the head of the critical care units at Regional Hospital. Nurse A has jurisdiction over the Cardiac Surgery Intensive Care Unit, the regular surgery's ICU and the Neonatal ICU. She has sufficient years behind her as a heart patient

care nurse to answer my questions. My CSICU stay was four days, but I knew others had much longer stays with more complications.

Nurse A and I met and talked in Regional Hospital's cafeteria over tinkling Christmas music and lunchroom chatter. What follows is the gist of our conversation, with me asking questions and Nurse A answering.

Suppose I came into the Emergency Room some night with indications of heart trouble, what would be my expectations?

After initial EKG tests confirmed a heart attack, you'd be rushed immediately to the catheterization lab (step two in my journey).

If they found you could be treated with a stent, they would do that. But if a stent or stents were not going to be able to solve the problem, you would have been brought to the CSICU for stabilization and had a consult with Dr. S, the full-time cardio-thoracic surgeon. Others can be called in if he's off-duty, but he's the main guy.

If Dr. S thought there was a need for an emergency surgery, we would have prepped you and got you into the operating room. The determination might be made on the basis of a more detailed electrocardiogram (also known as an ECG or EKG) that might indicate a STEMI[15] (pronounced "stemmy"), which is the term cardiologists use to refer to a classic heart attack.

---

15. A ST-Elevation Myocardial Infarction, more commonly known as a heart attack.

This was new jargon to me, and she explained that the graphical output of the EKG has certain phases lettered for easy reference. You've probably seen the spiky output of an EKG reading. The peaks and valleys are lettered P, Q, R, S, T and U.

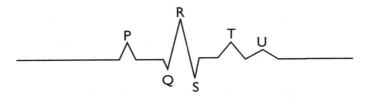

The S-T segment refers to what is typically the flat portion of the reading between heartbeats, but during a heart attack, that section will appear abnormally elevated. In this way, the EKG reading can visually indicate an ST-elevation myocardial infarction, meaning there's an occlusion somewhere in the arteries feeding your heart.

If you had a STEMI, you need surgery soon, better yet, right now.

I had a four-day stay, but is there a normal length of time for a hospital stay induced by a heart attack?

Typically, if a patient comes in as an outpatient, after surgery you'd come to the CSICU for post-op recovery. You might expect a five-day stay in our ward and a transfer to rehab for about a week after that.

So, normal for a CABG is five days in the CSICU and then about a week of rehab? Ten days? For someone who is uninsured, wouldn't that constitute an economic hazard that could ruin a family's economic future?

Yes, that would be a typical stay for someone who came in based on indications from an EKG. And it certainly could be financially crippling for a family that was uninsured.

What differentiated my four-day stay from this typical scenario?

Well, you're probably active at home (yes), and you probably did what you were told. You also did what the nurses asked. (I tried.)

There are two things that prolong a stay. One is, if you weren't active before, you're not likely to be active now. Getting out of bed or getting out of a chair with a weak heart takes a lot of energy. It's not just, "Oh, my gosh! I'm a little weak." Now you have a broken sternum and, when you're trying to move, it hurts. Those people who weren't active before aren't going to get up—they don't tend to get that needed movement.

Increased activity in that first 24 hours literally changes everything. Getting up drains the fluids out of the chest into the chest tubes. Even though they are the cause of most post-op pain, chest tubes are essential. Draining the chest cavity is a necessary part of the

healing process. The drainage is monitored for how much fluid is being produced and how clear it is.

The second thing that indicates how long your stay might be is how well you follow directions. When I tell you, "You have to get out of bed," you have to get out of bed. You need to have the gumption to get up and move, even if it hurts. Some patients feel a sense of victimhood and think, *I can't do that, I just had heart surgery*. They don't realize how much better they are going to feel after the surgery, how much more energy they are going to have.

You need to understand going into the surgery that *it's all about you*. If you get up and walk every day, if you ask to walk, if you sit up in the chair, if you don't ask to go right back to bed—these simple things can reduce your stay. And you need to use the incentive spirometer as much as you can. Don't wait for the nurse to tell you to use it.

That's a good quote. "It's all about you."

It's absolutely true. It's up to the patient to be involved in their healing. I've had some patients ask me, "Could you lift my arm for me?" *No!* You lifted it before you had surgery. You need to do it now; you have to get over the pain. And if you are in pain, don't be a hero. Take the medicines.

If you had a good nurse, she'll anticipate when she's going to get you out of bed and maybe up your morphine prior to getting you up, so you can do it

with less discomfort. (I had to agree, I had excellent nursing care.)

A little more serious case. If I had the "fall on the floor with a heart attack and someone finds me just in time" scenario and I've come in on an ambulance sometime later with a damaged heart, what might be an expected outcome?

That's going to be a pretty long stay. You probably need ten days to a few weeks in the CSICU, and *then* go to rehab at a long-term acute care center where you'll get better rehabilitation because there may be multiple traumas to treat.

If your heart has been damaged for even a short while, you probably have also damaged your lungs from lack of oxygen. The heart is the pump that keeps everything else going. So that gets fixed first, but you're going to need longer term care to repair those lungs.

Or you may have liver damage or will be having problems with your blood pressure.

So, the other patients in the unit that I saw simply lying there for days at a time—those critical care patients... Are they in a medically induced coma?

Occasionally, but those are usually only for patients who are on breathing tubes. There's that lung damage! Once the breathing tubes are out, we need to talk with these patients.

Other than "the healing is all about you," do you have any succinct advice for the individual or family that's facing one of these procedures?

A support system is important, and you have to take your meds. Some of the repeats we get, the patients that are back with complications after discharge, they don't take their meds when they go home. You'll be on anti-biotics; you need to take those.

Ask questions. If you don't understand what's being said, ask for more explanation. You may be still partially on pain meds, so make sure your support group understands what's being required of you.

Healing really is about you. Make sure you understand what is expected in terms of follow-up, and then follow up. Go to those appointments.

Make sure you go for a walk every day. If you have PT scheduled, do what they say.

You can't get well if you don't participate in your recovery. We can't bring you healing. We can give you the tools to get well, but we can't make you well. That's on you.

Then there are simple things, like washing your hands. If you go home with a fresh scar over your sternum or your chest tube openings, you can come back with infections if you don't wash your hands.

Take your showers, perform your self-care, make sure you're eating right. Then there are ileuses, which are intestinal obstructions—between the pain meds

and the trauma, the bowel backs up. You need to walk to help get things moving.

Keep your salt intake low for the first month or two.

Use the incentive spirometer to reduce the chances of pneumonia. Pneumonia is a big complication. So, use the incentive spirometer for several weeks to help clear the lungs of liquid and help restore tissues that have been affected by the incidental handling during surgery. You don't want to take deep breaths because it hurts to breathe, so the incentive spirometer helps get that lung capacity back. The spirometer also helps to remove any lingering anesthesia.

At the end of my conversation with Nurse A, I thanked her. The information she shared is very helpful.

Chapter 11

You Bet Your Life

A T THE TIME OF THIS WRITING, three months after the surgery, I still go to wellness classes at a gym with physical therapists on hand. The easy part was having the surgery. The almost-easy part was being sentenced to an easy chair for a month. The hard part will be not succumbing to my prior lifestyle again.

We related to Dr. S that I had lost a little over 10 lbs after the surgery. He nodded; that was about right. But he cautioned it can easily come right back. And *that* is the big problem. Both before and after surgery, there was and is that balance of diet and exercise that *should have been* maintained and should forever *continue to be* maintained.

I was not good at it before, hence my 234-lbs average weight for the past several years. I'm not sure what my post-surgery survival chances will be if I return to the fast food nation. The choices out there are not good, and the advertised specials are obnoxiously bad. Tacos

wrapped in cheese burritos, triple burgers, and triple-cheese Baconators! Really?

I know they have a profit motive and market research behind providing and shamelessly promoting 1,150-calorie sandwiches, but *you* don't have to go there anymore. The marketing professionals for all those fast food outlets are being paid to convince you to make bad choices, to fatten your arteries, to kill yourself.

So, to you, my reader, the challenge is made; the gauntlet is thrown down. The next time you go into a fried chicken palace, are you going for the 12-wing special with their secret sauce? Check the fat and sodium content and just say, "no."

Will you opt for the three-piece southern-fried special with mashed potatoes and brown gravy? Or will you consider the broiled white meat diced over a salad? *That* is a choice you can live with.

If you should decide on Italian food, great decision; I love the stuff too. Alfredo sauce? Not so good a choice as a tomato-based alternative. Butter slathered garlic bread sticks are also not so good. And Tuesday's endless pasta night? Really not good.

The choices are all out there and they are all yours. Thick crust vs. thin crust? What about a crust made of cauliflower? I've tried a few of those... With the marinara and additional items, it's a better choice than a thick crust Sicilian with three meats and cheeses.

It's about your choices. Is your seafood going to be deep-fried, breaded, broiled or baked? How about that sub? A foot-long or half that?

Eating on the road? Most major food stores have deli sections with pre-made salads. Many have small dining areas so you don't have to try to eat while driving. Slow down, and enjoy the meal. You might get back 15 minutes later than you'd planned, but your vascular system will love you for it.

Each of those choices is a roll of the dice, and the game is called "You Bet Your Life."

According to the Center for Disease Control, about 610,000 people die of heart disease in the U.S. every year, or about one-fourth of all deaths. Nearly 735,000 Americans have a heart attack every year, of which 525,000 are first-timers and 210,000 are recidivists (repeat offenders).

Look back at that math: 735,000 heart attacks, 610,000 deaths. The implication for me is that there is not a good survival rate.

Do you have the primary risk factors? High blood pressure, high cholesterol, or a history of smoking? Tell me you're not *still* smoking!

Some of the other big ones to check off:

- Diabetes
- Overweight or obese
- Poor diet
- Physically inactive
- Excessive alcohol consumption

I'll stop preaching. But are you in my club? Are you one of the pear-shaped wonders with a belt size in the

mid to upper 30s or, if you're a lady, do you shop in the plus sizes?

Then, please take note. I'm not body shaming here, just advising you to stop kidding yourself. You're inviting your body down that very expensive road to an emergency visit to the cardiac operating theater, where you are going to have the leading role. STEMIs aren't for everyone in the plus range, but you are inviting diabetes, and that's no fun either.

I was lucky—extremely so. A fortunate series of events led me to that operating room as one of the over 800,000 CABG operations that isn't one of the 735,000 heart attacks.

As I mentioned in the early chapters, an incredulous me took the advice of my nurse practitioner to seek further testing. I had been kidding myself. I ate crap on the road. I took side trips through the drive-thru for milkshake happy hour. I took advantage of the supersized peanut butter cups. I let food, and unhealthy food at that, provide solace to some sense of not quite being satisfied with the world or my place in it.

There are other cures for depression or frustration or anxiety that don't cause heart disease and that don't include in their ultimate cure a life-ending heart attack. But it's your life to gamble with. I hope you'll make better choices. If you start now, you might not need that bankruptcy-risking surgery. You might live to tell about it.

I met a friend of mine a few years ago who used to be in the pear-shaped club with me. When we spoke

recently, he was about thirty pounds lighter and nimble on his feet. I asked if he was okay. Cancer can do that to a person, as can diabetes. He said he'd been given a diagnosis of being pre-diabetic and took stock of his life. He began walking a lot and watching his diet. Two years later, he was down thirty-five pounds and had a clean bill of health.

So, final thoughts.

- Get a checkup, with an EKG. Ask your physician if you should get a coronary stress test.
- Start making better choices. Don't bet with your life.
- If you have a friend or loved one in similar straits, over forty, pear-shaped or larger, give them this book.

Epilogue

IF YOU'VE BOUGHT OR BEEN GIFTED this book because you are facing a cardiac bypass surgery of your own, take heart. Literally. You will feel a lot better afterward. You will have more energy, vitality and, if that's not important enough, added years to your life. You may not have noticed becoming more tired or winded after short periods of exercise. You may, like me, have attributed lower energy levels to the aging process. I'm now sixty-nine. I assumed I had less energy simply because I was out of shape and older.

The fact was, at rest, I had plenty of blood supply for sitting, simply moving around the house, or other light activities. But the stress test proved medically that I could not sustain prolonged heavy exertions, like raking the lawn or extended uphill hiking. I'm actually surprised that one of my hikes in the Carolina mountains or around Mt. Rainier didn't kill me. Certainly, a heart attack in those remote locations could have been fatal.

This addendum to my story might have been included in the Complications chapter, but I need to share this additional section.

For several months after discharge, I had been going to the Wellness Center three times a week, but at eight months, I joined a traditional gym. The lack of machines in the Wellness Center and the often fully-booked sessions made it hard to do anything but cardio. I still wanted to regain or at least maintain upper body, core and leg strength as I moved on.

On the second visit to the new gym, my trainer was taking me through some exercises and "working me," as I think back on it, to see what I could handle. I had by then told him of the CABG procedure over eight months prior. At one point, I found myself sitting on a bench and hearing my trainer asking repeatedly:

"Are you OK?"

"Are you with me?"

"Bruce, are you alright?"

Slowly, foggily, I realized I wasn't. I'd passed out. Only for thirty seconds, but I had fainted from lack of blood supply. This caused me some worry. I had been somewhat dehydrated (not good) and a little sleep deprived (also not good), but I had severe second thoughts about my ability to carry on.

I called for an appointment with Dr. P and was able to meet with his ARNP in a few weeks. That led to

another stress test and an almost immediate appointment for a second catheterization.

It was explained that, this time, they would go in through my groin rather than my wrist in anticipation of the insertion of a stent if blockages were found. I hadn't gotten precise information on the results of the stress test, but the catheterization would confirm the status of the bypass locations.

As I watched the images on the fluoroscope, I watched as blood inserted into the descending arteries seemed to backwash out of the aorta, not into the fine tree-like branching pattern I expected of blood spreading out into heart muscle. It was confirmed: two of the bypasses had collapsed and were no longer functioning. The native vessels, the ones that were initially noted as up to 80% blocked, were doing all the work.

Dr. P proceeded to install two stents. One in the artery that had not been addressed in the surgery and one in one of the native arteries that had been bypassed. This procedure is called a percutaneous coronary intervention (PCI). The stents I received were drug-eluting stents (DES). Literature suggests that these are more common now, for good reason.

Platelets are not your friend at this point. Used by your body to stop bleeding, they would normally attack and attach to a new stent, causing more of a blockage, adding to plaque buildup. The drug coating on the DES will inhibit that tendency for the first several weeks after being implanted, and your new prescription for

a blood thinner like Plavix or Brilinta will continue to protect you with the addition of a daily aspirin.

My understandable reaction to all this was to be disappointed, upset and concerned. I'd gone through a pretty strenuous experience for such a small return. One of the three initial bypass grafts was still working, but two had failed at some time afterward; no telling when. I scheduled follow-ups with both my cardiologist and surgeon to find out what exactly happened. Their reporting clarified that the two grafts from my veins were the two that failed. The graft from my mammary artery was still functional.

Checking professional literature, I find that up to 15% of vein grafts can fail within the first 12 months. Up to 50% could fail within ten years. But, even knowing that, for patients like me with several sites needing bypass grafts, multiple CABGs are the recommended strategy.

Post-stent life will include a continuing regimen of blood thinners. I can accept that; I just need to be much more cautious when doing things that might nick or cut me. Blood thinners and aspirin will make stopping any bleeding more difficult. Your doctor will also caution you against certain procedures like major dental work and colonoscopies. Bleeding from either of these would be problematic.

My surgeon, Dr. S, indicated there are no known indicators as to what kind of patients might be more susceptible than others to failure of grafted veins, a.k.a. saphenous vein grafts (SVGs). So, I'm looking forward

to a final round on the catheterization table to get the last two sites repaired. Here are some of the benefits I'm hoping for:

- I get a final sense of closure, knowing the titanium alloy stents cannot collapse.
- I can finally experience, hopefully, more strenuous activities—get back to the gym, play with my kayak at some remove from civilization—without worrying overly much about having a STEMI.

I say that because my diet is slowly working. I hit a plateau at 220 lbs, but eventually worked through it. I hit another at 210, and I've finally punched through that one.

It is not an easy thing; I will warn you. It simply is not an easy thing to regard some of your favorite foods as poison. But there it is. Fatty meats, cheeses (and I love cheeses), milkshakes and custard ice creams, sugar and cream cheese icing. Fried foods of all description are on that list.

I'll stop hitting you over the head about diet, but with the food change, there's exercise. Remember LDLs and HDLs? The LDLs are the ones from diet, the ones that will lead to plaque buildup. HDLs are the ones that come from exercise. They help control the bad behavior of the LDLs. So, I exercise to exorcise the LDLs via my liver.

Like I said, you are not going to fix this situation with surgery and a pill. You are the one in charge.

According to the American Heart Association, about 20% of heart attack patients 45 and older will have a second attack. I suspect failure to adopt healthy eating habits and failure to exercise are leading contributors to that statistic.

I hope my account of my experiences will shed some light on what you might expect from the CABG procedure and the recovery period.

The salient lesson for me was best summarized by Nurse A. "Healing is all about you."

Actively participating, proactively working to pay attention, exercising and practicing the best possible post-op hygiene will limit the expense of your hospital stay, make your post-discharge experience more comfortable, and dramatically reduce the chances of having a repeat engagement in the CSICU.

Thank you for reading *Welcome to the Zipper Club*. If you've enjoyed reading this book, please leave a review on your favorite review site. It helps me reach more readers who may benefit from the information provided herein.

Acknowledgments

First of all, I need to thank Kathy Odham for her initial recognition that I might have more serious problems than simple water retention. Her insight put me on the road to having my heart overhauled.

My next logical expression of appreciation goes to the professionals at the Capital Cardiology Associates, especially Drs. Pandit, who diagnosed my need for a coronary artery bypass graft, and Dr. Jeffery Snyder, who installed those said grafts.

Proceeding chronologically… Kudos to the professional nursing staff and support team at Tallahassee's Capital Regional Medical Center. As many of these folk are traveling nurses, some are not there now, but lend their TLC to patients elsewhere.

My wife, Christine Chiricos, and daughter, Sarah Mullane (who has a BSN in nursing), provided the best home care support team I could have hoped for. Recovery wasn't always easy, but they helped smooth the bumps.

And for making the idea of this book, with its very rough start, something worth sharing, I thank Tara Alemany and Mark Gerber at Emerald Lake Books. They have brought *Welcome to the Zipper Club* to the world in more than its initial amateurish presentation. Their insight and professionalism are obvious in its editing, formatting and design.

Thank you, all.

About the Author

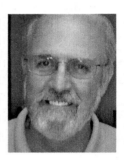

LIKE MANY PEOPLE, Bruce Ballister's youth as a skinny kid did not presage his obese adulthood. Although slender through high school, the U.S. Army and college life, his waist size grew from 26" to 30" by the age of thirty, finally stabilizing at 38" in his 60s.

Shortly before his bout with heart disease, he retired from a full-time professional life and started considering the next pants size up.

His plans to pursue a second career as a science fiction author and occasional consultant were sidetracked when a surprising interview at an annual physical threatened his very life.

The news of his heart disease came as a shock. His search for understanding what to expect from quadruple bypass surgery and recovery led to the writing of this book.

Bruce's hope is to provide you with the information he looked for, but couldn't find. He has drawn on his actual experiences, augmented with research and interviews with a few of the real healthcare professionals he came in contact with on his journey.

He is happy to report that he is well on his way to pursuing his second career as a happier, healthier and size-34″ retiree, enjoying his science fiction writing and part-time consulting.

If you're interested in having Bruce come speak to your group or organization about preventative health measures or heart health, either online or in person, you can contact him at emeraldlakebooks.com/ballister.

Recommended Resources

Centers for Disease Control and Prevention. "Defining Adult Overweight and Obesity."
elbks.com/zipcdc.

UpToDate. "Patient Education: Coronary Artery Bypass Graft Surgery (Beyond the Basics)."
elbks.com/zipuptodate.

Johns Hopkins Medicine. "Coronary Artery Bypass Graft Surgery."
elbks.com/ziphopkins.

Honor Health. "Coronary Artery Bypass Graft Surgery."
elbks.com/ziphonor.

National Center for Biotechnology Information. "Saphenous vein graft failure and clinical outcomes: Toward a surrogate end point in patients following coronary artery bypass surgery?"
elbks.com/zipncbi.

US Cardiology Review. "Current Thinking In Acute Congestive Heart Failure And Pulmonary Edema." elbks.com/zipuscard.

For more great books, please visit us at
emeraldlakebooks.com.

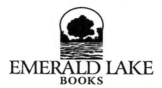

Made in the USA
Middletown, DE
04 October 2020

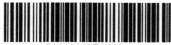